FIT AT MID-LIFE

SAMANTHA BRENNAN
& TRACY ISAACS

FIT AT MID-LIFE

A Feminist
Fitness
Journey

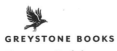

GREYSTONE BOOKS
Vancouver/Berkeley

Greystone Books Ltd.
www.greystonebooks.com

Cataloguing data available from Library
and Archives Canada
ISBN 978-1-77164-167-8 (pbk.)
ISBN 978-1-77164-168-5 (epub)

Editing by Stephanie Fysh
Proofreading by Stefania Alexandru
Cover and text design by Naomi MacDougall
Cover photograph by iStockphoto.com
Printed and bound in Canada on ancient-forest-friendly
paper by Friesens

We gratefully acknowledge the support of the Canada
Council for the Arts, the British Columbia Arts Council,
the Province of British Columbia through the Book
Publishing Tax Credit, and the Government of Canada for
our publishing activities.

Canadä

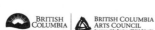

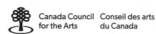

For the ever-growing community of fit feminists who read and comment at Fit Is a Feminist Issue. You inspire us daily.

CONTENTS

Acknowledgements

THE BOOK grew out of the blog *Fit Is a Feminist Issue,* which we started to document our Fittest by 50 Challenge. We want to thank the blog readers, commenters, and guest bloggers who have embraced and advanced the conversation about an alternative, more feminist, approach to fitness. Special thanks go to regular contributors and frequent guest bloggers: Natalie Hébert, Catherine Womack, Cate Creede, Martha Muzychka, Audrey Yap, Christine Daigle, Catherine Hundleby, Michelle Goodfellow, Stephanie Keating, Rebecca Kukla, Jessica Schagerl, Kim Solga, Susan Tarshis, Chloe Wall, Elan Paulson, and Tracy de Boer. A warm shout-out and high-five go to Caitlin Constantine, our faster, younger fit feminist friend and sister-blogger, a formidable athlete, who forged the path on *Fit and Feminist* with the spot-on tagline "Because it takes strong women to smash the patriarchy." And the blog wouldn't be the same without Jean, from Cycle Write Blog, who comments on just about every new post (and there are a lot of new posts). We extend thanks also to Aviva Shiller, our research assistant and guest poster. We owe a huge debt of gratitude to Lisa Adams of the Garamond Agency, who worked closely with us to give shape to our book; to Nancy Flight of Greystone Books, who helped bring our project to fruition; and to Pam Robertson, whose smart editing decisions resulted in a much better book than we would have been able to produce without her.

Sam also thanks coach Chris Helwig and his thriving community of women cyclists; the members of the Aiki Budo Centre; Dave Henry and Jennifer Broxterman of CrossFit London and NutritionRx; the women of the London Rowing Club; Jeff; Sarah and Kathleen; her children, Mallory, Gavin, and Miles; her mother, Kathleen; and all of her cycling friends, especially her fellow participants in the Friends for Life Bike Rally.

Tracy also thanks Balance Point Triathlon coach Gabbi Whitlock; the early-morning swimming crew (especially in lane 2) at the London Centre Branch Y; Karen Major of Yoga Centre London; the London, Ontario, Running Room Run Club and clinics; running buddies Anita Kothari and Julie Riley; Daphne Gray-Grant (The Publication Coach); her parents, Ray and Norma, who are role models for vitality and active living; her step-daughter, Ashley Joy; and Renald.

PART ONE

Feminist Fitness and Fittest by 50

ONE

Introducing the Fittest by 50 Challenge

WE CAN sometimes forget that we won't live forever, but when our age is about to click over from one decade to the next, many of us make big life changes, often committing to new health regimes with the hope of aging well, if not preserving our youth. The mid-life decade birthdays—40, 50, 60—start to loom about a year or two before we get to them. People like to view these milestones as calls to action. That's when we start new diets or ramp up those occasional runs into more regular training. There's even a name for these individuals: 9-enders. Studies show that when 9-enders run a marathon, they do better than people two years younger or older. The spectre of a new decade spurs them to train harder.

We were hired just one year apart (1992 and 1993) into the Department of Philosophy at Western University in London, Ontario. We discovered many similarities in our backgrounds and world views. Both of us had immigrated to Canada with our families as young children. We'd both gone to the U.S. to do our philosophy PhDs. We shared research interests in ethics and feminist philosophy. And we'd both been born in 1964, less than a month apart. Through countless coffees, lunches, walks, and chats in the department, we've had a more than 20-year conversation about dieting, fitness, and the social pressure on women to see these in relation to only one goal: getting thin. But diets don't work in the long run (sorry, they just don't), and there are lots of other, more self-nurturing and empowering reasons to play sports and get active.

On the eve of our 48th birthdays, as 50 came into view, we set ourselves this challenge: by the time we turned 50, we would be the fittest we've ever been in our lives. We called it our Fittest by 50 Challenge (FB50, for short). To document our challenge and to invite others to join our conversation, we launched the blog Fit, Feminist, and (almost) Fifty.

We expected our friends and relatives to read it. We could not have predicted the blog's impact. It started off small—a few hundred readers in the first month, a few hundred more in the second. In the sixth month, the blog registered over 20,000 hits. By the end of the seventh month, that had more than doubled, to over 44,000. We'd struck a chord.

Our challenge had begun when, right before her 48th birthday, Sam posted this on social media: "As I approach the two-year countdown to 50 (I turn 48 at the end of this summer) I'd like to set an ambitious fitness goal. Roughly, I'd like to be the *most fit* I've ever been at 50." A long thread of comments ensued. People had all sorts of views about what markers would make good evidence of "most fit." Speed? Heart rate? Increased distance in running or cycling? Body composition?

Tracy joined in the challenge and we launched the blog to give us some accountability, with a more public goal. At the same time, it presented a great opportunity for us to continue the conversation with a larger community. We would blog about our efforts to reach our Fittest by 50 (FB50) goal, and along the way, develop our feminist approach to fitness. We wanted to write for a general audience of women and to offer them an alternative way to think about their fitness goals, divorced from the cultural obsession with looking a certain way. We were sick of that perspective, and we guessed we weren't alone.

Physical activity is a tremendous source of joy for both of us. The blog attracted like-minded readers as well as those who were ready to try a new way. Many women have been put off by the whole idea of fitness and are fed up with the regular messages they receive from fitness gurus, books, and blogs about how to lose weight on restrictive diets. And why shouldn't we be? Our cultural bias favours looks over physical strength, health, and fitness—and sets most of us up to fail. If you're like us, you are tired of hearing about long cardio sessions and light weights. And you're even more weary of the sea of pink that dominates women's fitness: pink shoes, pink yoga clothes, pink running skirts, pink stability balls, pink dumbbells. Enough!

We are living proof that there is another way.

It's not easy to reject the strong cultural messages about losing weight and the obligation to diet that bombard us daily from all directions. Even when we become aware that dieting for weight loss isn't working for us, it's tough to resist the magnetic force of the idea that if we could just lose a few pounds, we'd be okay. We also need to get past the view that exercise and physical activity are joyless duties that we need to undertake to keep our unwieldy bodies in check.

There are lots of good reasons to resist the mainstream view. Reason number one: Why miss out on the fun you could have? We can reclaim play in our adult lives. Reason number two: Medical and health research has shown over and over again the slim odds of losing weight and keeping it off over the long term. So let's set that aside and look for other sources of motivation. That's where fun comes into the picture. According to Dr. Michelle Segar, director of the Sport, Health and Activity Research and Policy Center at the University of Michigan, fun motivates us more. It turns out that people who work out for health and weight-loss reasons typically work out less than people who do it because it feels good. And an active lifestyle gives us energy and strength as we age and becomes a whole new source of fun and friendship.

Within six months we had a steadily growing community of readers regularly coming to the blog and leaving their thoughts in the comments. It became clear to us that there just aren't many places out there where you can find people asking questions that challenge commonly held views about what it means to get and be fit. What if you could be tremendously fit and healthy yet not lose weight? It's a rare corner of the internet where you find anyone who takes that possibility seriously. And how often do we even see older athletes represented in the mainstream sports and fitness media? Our blog made room for (and now, renamed Fit Is a Feminist Issue, continues to make space for) these alternative kinds of conversations.

What to Expect from This Book

As you read, you'll notice three different things going on in this book. One is the thread of our personal narratives—our stories of our individual experiences in undertaking our Fittest by 50 Challenge, each told from our own perspective. These are first-person accounts, told from the "I" point of view, and appear as distinct chapters at the end of each of the book's four parts. The other chapters take up different issues in and aspects of fitness and paint them with a feminist brush. Sometimes we offer social commentary; sometimes we give overviews of the facts and latest research. When you read those chapters, you'll hear the voice of a unified "we," but when we use our own experiences as examples, we talk about "Tracy" and "Sam" so you don't get confused about which of us we're referring to. Finally, even though this is not a how-to book, we do have tips, strategies, and thoughts that we'd like to share with you, things that might help you as you think through the pursuit of fitness in your own life. You'll run into these offerings all over the place, and every chapter other than the personal narratives ends with "Take it away...," where we remind you of the chapter's main message, and "Try this...," where we encourage you to give something a go.

Most of all, if you're frustrated with the dominant narrative about women's fitness, we hope *Fit at Mid-Life* inspires you to join us and the many women we know who have reclaimed fitness on their own terms.

Take it away...

Instead of viewing a 9-ender year—or any looming new year—with dread, we can use it to embark on an exciting challenge. Using fun as a motivator and setting aside the idea that the number on the scale is the most important thing, we can redefine fitness in our middle years. As women who have been bombarded with all sorts of messages about how we're supposed to look, let's use this time of life to challenge ourselves in new, exciting ways that defy expectations.

Try this....

Is there a sport you've always wanted to try or a physical activity you've wanted to take up? Why not use your next birthday as an occasion to branch out and do it? You could even hire a trainer or expert for an intro session—it'd be the perfect gift from someone special, or to yourself.

TWO
Older and Wiser

Aging also helps us grow into ourselves. We start to know what we like and don't like. We stop giving a fuck what other people think of us. Imagine, young'uns, a world where you just don't give a shit about looking stupid or what your friends think or falling down in public or impressing the Joneses or having to go along with the crowd to do things you hate. Imagine how awesome that would be. The liberation. The joyous freedom. The glorious sense of possibility. Well, if you're lucky, that's what getting older is.
KRISTA SCOTT DIXON[1]

DO YOU have to be young to be fit? *We* don't believe that, but judging by media representations of fitness, you might think so. Magazines and websites devoted to fitness typically feature images of very young men and women (mostly also white and non-disabled and already pretty fit-looking). There's a popular phenomenon called *fitspiration,* or *fitspo,* that depicts these types of images, sometimes with accompanying sayings like "You don't get what you wish for, you get what you work for" or "Don't wait for the inspiration, be the inspiration." This is supposed to inspire "ordinary people" to go out and get active so they too can look young and lean and thin and beautiful. Sometimes fitness and other advertising does feature older people—but it's always an uber-fit, bright-teethed salt-and-pepper couple who appear to have retired early to kayak the rugged coast.

While the research makes clear that we benefit from starting a program of exercise, especially resistance training, at any age, the exclusion from fitness images of older people we can relate to (rather than feel intimidated by) makes the first steps harder to take. For the person who wants to embark on working out in mid-life and beyond, the road can be lonely. The numbers of older people taking part in most recreational sports are strikingly low. Older women are especially scarce. Maybe this very thing has kept *you* from venturing into activities that appeal to you.

We need to combat the view that only youthful bodies are worthy of being seen. Fear of "looking foolish" keeps many older women away from physical activity altogether. And aging is particularly tough on women when society puts such a high value on appearance and when beauty seems inextricably linked with youth. Like Bette Davis says, "Old age is not for sissies," but an active lifestyle makes mid-life and beyond much easier.

As we age, the gap between the physically fit and capable and those who lead sedentary lifestyles grows wider and the health implications become more serious. But it's not an insurmountable problem... if we can find ways to make physical activity more accessible and attractive to everyone.

Use It or Lose It: Is Aging a Lifestyle Choice?

As more people stay physically active into their senior years, people are smashing age group records in almost every sport and fitness endeavour, from rock climbing to running, rowing to weightlifting. The new super fit seniors have even made their way into mainstream television: the British reality show *Are You Fitter Than a Pensioner?* pits super fit 70-somethings from California against out-of-shape British young people. Of course these seniors are the exception to the norm, but it goes to show that vitality isn't necessarily tied to age.

Recent research measured older athletes' ages in fitness terms and showed some amazing results. As a result of cardiovascular health, the fitness age of super fit participants in the U.S's National Senior Games is as much as 25 years lower than their chronological age, says the University of Maryland's Dr. Pamela Peeke, a triathlete who started running at age 40.[2] She measured the competitors' fitness age with a specialized calculator designed by Norwegian researchers.

At the same time, other research shows that people of the same chronological age can age at radically different rates. Genetics play a role, but some of the differences relate to fitness and physical activity. A study of nearly one thousand 38-year-olds found that while most had biological ages close to their actual age, others were far younger or older. Researchers used 18 markers, including blood pressure, organ function, and metabolism, to assess the health-adjusted age of each of the participants. Their results ranged from a biological age of 26, at the young end of the spectrum, to 61, at the older end.

As Duke University's Daniel Belsky commented at the time, "The overwhelming majority are biologically in their mid-40s or younger, but there are a handful of cases who are in pretty bad shape. In the future, we'll come to learn about the different lives that fast and slow ageing people have lived."[3]

So it looks as if we have some choice about how we age, and that exercise has tremendous protective effects on our health even as we get into our later years. It would be misleading to say that we can stop aging altogether by staying active, but if we reject the idea that our year of birth should dictate the activities we enjoy, we can choose to age well. So go ahead! Take up mountain biking. Learn to downhill ski. Join that tai chi class. Sign up for West Coast swing dancing.

Exercise doesn't just help physical health. For mental health and cognitive capacity, there's a good case for saying that you ought to put down that Sudoku puzzle and hop on your bike. A University of Texas at Austin study published in the journal *Medicine & Science in Sports & Exercise* in 2015 showed that those who regularly exercise perform better on memory-related tests and have higher scores in terms of cognitive functioning.[4] The findings from this study suggest that middle-aged endurance athletes not only have better cardiovascular function and health, but also have enhanced cognitive performance, particularly in the domains linked with age-related cognitive decline and impairment. Dr. Martha Pyron, a co-author of the study, concludes that "habitual aerobic exercise ameliorates vascular health, an effect which may further translate into improved cognitive performance."

Gretchen Reynolds, in her book on exercise science, *The First 20 Minutes,*[5] makes the interesting point that aging, in some respects, might be something we're *choosing* to do. Reynolds asks, what exactly is the connection between exercise and aging? In what she calls "the old view," muscle loss and a decline in aerobic capacity are inevitable with old age. The assumption is that starting in our 40s, we slow down with age and become more frail. But new research suggests the connections may run the other way: we get slower and more frail because we stop moving. Older athletes get slower and less strong not because they're older, but rather because they train less than younger athletes.

We age because we stop moving, and that is a choice we make. Intriguing idea? You bet. It gives us some control: if we choose differently, if we continue or increase our physical activity, we can fend off the effects of aging. Of course, lots of factors contribute to the aging process, but our activity level is one that many of us can control to at least some degree. It's worth reflecting on this on entering mid-life: Does the suggestion that we can choose how to age make you think differently about some of the decisions you might make for yourself?

Sam got a taste of the "use it or lose it" rule when she went to physio for an injured shoulder. In addition to providing her with a host of exercises, staff at the clinic complimented her for getting right back to Aikido and CrossFit. She shared with the physiotherapist the worry of friends and relatives that she ought to slow down while her shoulder healed, maybe even take time off from lifting weights and doing martial arts. Yeah, he replied, lots of people think that, and then they never regain the range of motion they had and it gets harder to go back to your usual physical activities. Keep moving, he said.

How to Age Better: Stop Caring about "Losing Your Looks"

What are the barriers to staying active or becoming active as we age? For many older women, it's a fear of not fitting in. And it's true that in some sports there just aren't that many older women. Sam regularly rides bikes with men in their 60s and 70s, but at 50, she's often the oldest woman.

There's also the focus on exercising for appearance—for getting or maintaining a thin or toned body, which can be tough for older women. The thought is, "I'm never going to look young again. Why bother?" A few recent studies show that women who care the most about their looks have the toughest time aging.

According to a 2014 study, the media plays a part in women's declining sense of self-worth as they age.[6] The older we get, the less "in line" we are with society's obsession with youthful appearance. For women whose appearance has been an important source of self-esteem, aging can take an especially brutal toll as they no longer see themselves as meeting expectations of attractiveness associated with being young.

Okay. We live a society in which a woman's worth is judged in terms of physical attractiveness and we all want to be valued and loved, so how do we navigate this minefield as we age? You know as well as we do that it's not a simple matter of choosing not to care. If you've invested lots of your own self-esteem in looking good, how can you move past that?

How about expanding the boundaries of beauty to include age diversity? Remind yourself of all the people you find beautiful who do not match society's standards of what counts. When you need to push past the idea that beauty ends at 30, 40, 50, or whatever silly age you have in mind, call up images of beautiful older people you admire.

We'd all do ourselves a big favour if we cared less than we do about beauty anyway. Many women seem *more* obsessed with clothes, hair, makeup, and so on as they age. They're worried about "letting themselves go." But caring more can set you up on an anxious, downward spiral. Let's care about things that matter much more than looks, things like character and having happy, healthy relationships.

Mid-life is the time to branch out and to put your self-esteem eggs in more than one basket. Look away from the mirror and reach out to find community and to find out that your body is made for a lot more than to be looked at. There's sheer joy in physical movement and achievement that has nothing to do with how you look.

We can care less about beauty and still care about looks. There may be a mainstream ideal beauty type, but at the same time we all have our own ideas about what looks good. No one needs everyone in the world to think her attractive. Most of us just want people, *particular* people, to find us attractive. But that's not capital B beauty. It doesn't make any sense to think about being attractive, period, from some non-relative point of view. What exactly would that mean? There is only "attractive to particular people." Different features draw in different people, just like people favour different body types. As cyclist Selene Yeager puts it, "If you're concerned about being 'unattractive' because you have big strong legs or broad shoulders, ask yourself 'unattractive to whom?' And maybe more importantly, 'Why do I want to be attractive to someone who isn't attracted to the real, active, bike-riding me?' "[7]

Why Bother? Aren't We All Going to Die Anyway?

Some people say that all this focus on mid-life exercise is just desperation, trying to fight off death. We hear it enough, and maybe you do too. Inevitably someone says, as if it never occurred to us, "You're just going to die anyway. Why work so hard? You can't cheat death, you know."

Someone we know uses the phrase "fighting off decrepitude." But remember, that's not inevitable. And that battle talk doesn't match our motivation, either. Age isn't the enemy that needs to be defeated. How about being the best 50-somethings we can be? Most active people in their 70s are as fit as those in their 50s. In a study of older cyclists, people aged 79 and people aged 55 showed little physical difference between one another if they maintained similar levels of exercise. Think about that for a minute. Isn't it an astonishing fact, one that defies most of our preconceptions about getting old?

We talked about aging *well*. But how about the idea that women ought to age "gracefully"? That there is some set of rules we ought to follow as the years catch up with us? That we're just too old to race our bikes, run marathons, colour our hair neon green, wear a bikini or a sleeveless shirt or low-rise jeans?

Cyclist Julie Lockhart starting riding and racing at age 70. Olga Kotelko started competing in track in her 70s and set all sorts of age-group records well into her 90s. Go ahead. Do the unexpected. Break a few rules. We can age well without slinking "gracefully" into the shadows like people expect us to. Another perk of aging: we can care less about what people think.

No one says we're going to live forever. Whether you think of it as sad, merciful, or just the unfettered truth, mortality is part of the human condition. But it's more than a little reassuring that older people can still have fun and defy social expectations about aging by riding their bikes. Let's keep the joy alive, even if that won't keep us alive forever. Three cheers for aging well!

What about Menopause?

When we hit menopause, our bodies start to change. It gets harder to lose weight, and the drop in estrogen means that body fat distributes differently. If you're there, you already know that fat settles around the belly. And your metabolism slows right down too. It's a double whammy for some of us—belly fat *and* a slower metabolism.

This leads to a spate of weight-loss advice for women in or approaching menopause. If menopausal women gain belly fat and their metabolisms slow down, they must be in a panic and want to lose weight! You need go no further than the Mayo Clinic website to find a 2016 article called "Menopause Weight Gain: Stop the Middle Age Spread."

It's no big surprise that the Mayo Clinic recommends that we eat less, move more: "Remember, successful weight loss at any stage of life requires permanent changes in diet and exercise habits. Take a brisk walk every day. Try a yoga class. Swap cookies for fresh fruit. Split restaurant meals with a friend. Commit to the changes and enjoy a healthier you!"

We say to this tired advice: "Yawn."

By all means, move more. But we can't say it enough: for most of us "eat less, move more" never worked. So why should we think that it transforms into a winning formula in menopause? How about not fixating on body weight quite so much and just doing things you love? Tracy hit menopause partway through the FB50 Challenge. If she'd set weight loss as part of her FB50 Challenge, she'd have had to quit before the end of it. She did some combination of running, swimming, biking, resistance training, and yoga just about every day, and her weight hovered within about two pounds of the same weight right through it. She didn't measure her body fat percentage, but she's convinced it didn't change either. Yet she had a blast and a leading online fitness age calculator reported that she reached the fitness level of someone younger than 20.[8]

Advice about avoiding menopausal weight gain by watching what you eat and focusing on eating less ushers in a new and alarming reality: the proliferation of eating disorders among women in mid-life.

The *Journal of Women & Aging* published a study of women and body satisfaction at mid-life and found that only 12.2% felt satisfied.[9] Cynthia Bulik published *Midlife Eating Disorders* in 2013 for "men and women in mid-life beyond, from all ethnic backgrounds," who "struggle with anorexia nervosa, bulimia nervosa, purging disorder, and binge eating disorder." Bulik points out that when we think of eating disorders most of us picture thin, white, upper-middle-class teenaged girls. But this assumption that only young people suffer these disorders renders less noticeable the equally alarming trend among older adults.

Regardless of body size, body weight, and body fat percentage, active women feel better about their bodies than inactive women. So if you're a menopausal woman who feels frustrated by weight gain or belly fat, you can feel better about yourself and your body if you take up a more active lifestyle.

Take it away...
Exercise and physical activity matter more than ever as we age—even if fitness culture includes us less and less. Let's make room for moving more and caring less about what others think.

Try this...
It's tough to flout the rules when you've spent a lifetime following them. Have you always wanted to try synchronized swimming or belly dancing (or anything else) but now worry that you're "too old" or it's too late? Says who? Try it.

THREE
Feminist Fitness Is for Everyone

FEMINIST FITNESS is for everyone. It's not just for women. For sure, strong, confident, capable women are good for all of us. They're great role models for children. They're contributing members of our communities. But a more inclusive approach to fitness wouldn't extend itself only to women. Though women will experience some of the challenges we raise uniquely or more intensely, men too can benefit from a more inclusive, joy-based approach to fitness.

While there's not one definition of feminism, the feminist principles that motivate *our* approach are equality and inclusivity. We regard these as important social justice values that go beyond sports and fitness to create better societies.

We like to imagine a world of sport and fitness where everyone is welcome, accepted, and encouraged, where people of all shapes, sizes, colours, genders, abilities, sexualities, and ages feel a sense of belonging and can participate without being judged.

We offer this book as an invitation of sorts, in the hopes that you will join us and the growing community of people who pursue fitness because of its potential to transform.

We want to highlight four ways feminist fitness can lead our own lives and to the lives of the people around us to flourish:

confidence and empowerment, happiness, body positivity, and agency.

We Can Do It! Confidence and Empowerment

The race T-shirt for the 2015 Niagara Women's Marathon has the word *Empowerment* across its front in bold yellow lettering. It's an oft-used, possibly even overused, word. But the fact is, empowerment and its close cousin, confidence, are feminist issues because there is a confidence gap. Men are way more confident than women in all sorts of ways. And because we live in a world where confidence takes people further than competence, that gap cashes out into all kinds of systemic advantages for men.

Katty Kay and Claire Shipman elaborate:

> Compared with men, women don't consider themselves as ready for promotions, they predict they'll do worse on tests, and they generally underestimate their abilities. This disparity stems from factors ranging from upbringing to biology.
>
> A growing body of evidence shows just how devastating this lack of confidence can be. Success, it turns out, correlates just as closely with confidence as it does with competence. No wonder that women, despite all our progress, are still woefully underrepresented at the highest levels. All of that is the bad news.[1]

So the bad news is, women haven't got as much confidence as men and that has a negative impact on where women get to in life. The good news, the authors go on to say, is that there are things that can change this. Finding ways for women to gain confidence—that is, ways to empower women—will take us that much closer to social equality. Participation in physical activity and sports, it turns out, is one of those ways.

Kay and Shipman describe U.S. research that shows that participation in sport alone has a positive impact on confidence, but also that girls tend to drop out of sports in high school:

Studies evaluating the impact of the 1972 Title IX legislation, which made it illegal for public schools to spend more on boys' athletics than on girls', have found that girls who play team sports are more likely to graduate from college, find a job, and be employed in male-dominated industries. There's even a direct link between playing sports in high school and earning a bigger salary as an adult. Learning to own victory and survive defeat in sports is apparently good training for owning triumphs and surviving setbacks at work. And yet, despite Title IX, fewer girls than boys participate in athletics, and many who do quit early. According to the Centers for Disease Control and Prevention, girls are still six times as likely as boys to drop off sports teams, with the steepest decline in participation coming during adolescence. This is probably because girls suffer a larger decrease in self-esteem during that time than do boys.

What a vicious circle: girls lose confidence, so they quit competing, thereby depriving themselves of one of the best ways to regain it.

If you're one of the women our age who had a not-so-great experience in sports as a girl, you might wonder whether you'd be a more confident athlete today if that had been different. And things *are* changing for girls and young women today. In many communities, soccer, hockey, rugby, and baseball are as available to girls as to boys. Based on what we know about the relationship between levels of confidence and participation in sports, these increased opportunities promise to usher in a more confident generation of young women.

It's encouraging to know that even as adults who missed these chances earlier in our lives, we can work on this. When we take up sports and physical activity, our confidence increases. After our FB50 Challenge, Tracy reflected on all the different things she'd done that, at the beginning, she would have thought impossible. Any distance of triathlon, running 10K, riding a road bike that she had to clip into, getting up in time to reach the edge of town for a 6 a.m. open water swim twice a week in the summer, training outside through the polar vortex of 2014—all impossible! But *not* impossible. Because Tracy did it.

If you struggle with low self-confidence, don't let it hold you back—you can cultivate a sense of confidence and empowerment by getting physically active.

Happiness, a Not-So-Elusive Goal

"Melancholy is incompatible with bicycling," wrote James Starrs in *The Literary Cyclist,* and while cycling may not be your thing, it's true that exercise has a tremendous effect on mood. Exercise helps with depression and anxiety, and along with getting enough sleep, it is the best thing you can do to lift your spirits.

Midway through the FB50 Challenge, Sam experienced the death of both of her parents-in-law, one to ALS and the other to a stroke, and she thought the whole thing might come off the rails. Instead, riding her bike and running in the woods with her dogs was about the only thing that kept her going through some very rough patches. She and her partner, Jeff, found long bike rides together to be the best therapy available. They rode their bikes a lot that awful summer, and Sam has no doubt that in the end it helped their moods.

It's lovely to arrive at work after walking or biking—there's the very nice gap between home and the office that helps keep a smile on your face. Exercising outdoors, it turns out, has double the benefits of indoor exercise. There are real mood and mental health benefits to spending time in nature, and studies show that women who exercise outside are more likely to stick with it.

Gretchen Reynolds, in a the *New York Times* column, writes, "In a number of recent studies, volunteers have been asked to go for two walks for the same time or distance—one inside, usually on a treadmill or around a track, the other outdoors. In virtually all of the studies, the volunteers reported enjoying the outside activity more and, on subsequent psychological tests, scored significantly higher on measures of vitality, enthusiasm, plea-sure and self-esteem and lower on tension, depression and fatigue after they walked outside."[2]

Research by a team at the Peninsula College of Medicine and Dentistry showed that exercising outdoors is associated with "greater feelings of revitalisation, increased energy and posi-tive engagement, together with decreases in tension, confusion, anger and depression."[3] We are just happier when we exercise out-side. Participants in studies of the benefits of outdoor exercise "also reported greater enjoyment and satisfaction with outdoor activity and stated that they were more likely to repeat the activ-ity at a later date."

And if you're interested in motivation for exercise, then look no further than the immediate mood boost. People who exer-cise for the immediate rewards of feeling better are more likely to exercise than those who do it for long-term health benefits. You've probably experienced it lots of times yourself—you debate with yourself about getting out of bed for that swim before work, and you stick with the plan. By the time you're in the pool, you're already feeling better. And by the time you hit the shower, you're practically singing, so happy you are that you went for it. Finish-ing a workout never leaves you regretting it.

Research shows that people whose goals are weight loss and better health exercise much less than those who do it for the mood boost or for the chance to connect with family and friends. Dr. Michelle Segar, director of the Sport, Health and Activity Research and Policy Center (SHARP) at the University of Michi-gan, says those of us who frame exercise as positive, restorative activity, because it makes us feel better, are more likely to get out there and do it.[4]

Rock It! On Exercise and Body Positivity

Work out because you love your body, not because you hate it, we say.

More than just inclusive, a feminist approach to fitness is also body positive. What does it mean to be body positive? At a minimum, it means that we don't come at fitness from a place of self-loathing. There's no fat-shaming and no thin-shaming in a feminist approach to fitness. A feminist approach to fitness instead means that we actively celebrate the incredible diversity in the human form. Think about movement and physical activity as a celebration of what our bodies can do.

We're not suggesting you start loving your body and *then* start working out. Being positive about the body you have can take work. If you're not there yet, it's not as if you can flick a switch overnight, from self-loathing one day to self-loving the next. Rather, make a start at getting active and go from there. Exercise and physical fitness can change our attitudes about our bodies. Women athletes, for example, report much higher levels of body self-esteem than non-athletes, and not because they look better. Among teenagers, sports participation has been found to be protective against a range of eating disorders and self-esteem issues. With eating disorders on the rise in women in mid-life, exercise might be protective for us as well.

What is true is that active women are more likely than inactive women to be happy with their bodies, even at the same size. A *Runner's World* headline a few years ago read "Few Middle-Aged Women Are Happy with Their Body Size: The Ones Most Likely to Be Are Highly Active." The article reported on the study in the *Journal of Women & Aging,* mentioned earlier, the one that found only 12.2% of older women were satisfied with their bodies. Exercise was part of what made the difference:

> Body satisfaction reflected considerable effort by the women to achieve and maintain rather than passive contentment, according to study authors. Satisfied women had lower BMI and exercised more than dissatisfied women, while weight monitoring and appearance-altering behaviors, such as cosmetic surgery, did not differ between the two groups.[5]

Cyclist Selene Yeager puts the connection between loving your body and being active this way: "Your body is the only one you've got. It's made to do things—like ride bikes and swing tennis racquets and hug people you love and jump for joy. It is to be lived through, not reserved for show like an empty, lifeless model home."[6]

Women of Action: On Exercise and Agency

Confidence and a sense of empowerment are great things, but getting physically active can create a different kind of internal shift, one that goes beyond the psychological. We begin to experience ourselves and our bodies differently. One way of putting it is that we gain a confident sense of ownership over our bodies—we gain a sense of our agency.

Feminists talk a lot about our embodied experience. All the triathlon training that Tracy undertook for the challenge altered the way she feels in her body, the way she occupies it. For the very first time in her life, she had (and continues to have) a sense of her physicality as belonging totally, 100%, to her.

When you get physically active, you own those activities—every endurance run, every early morning workout in the pool, every victory on the bike. They're yours. You do them for yourself. Not for us or for your parents or your partner or your kids or because someone else/society/your employer/Oprah thinks you should. Nope. None of that. No one would blink an eye if you never did any of this stuff again. And yet, if you've found those things you're passionate about, you do them anyway because they're things *you want to do.*

There's great power in that.

When Sam started training in martial arts, it changed the way she moved in the world and felt about her ability to stand her ground and defend herself. She is more confident, but it's not just that. She also has a much clearer sense of her boundaries and can move quickly when they're crossed. Among our community of guest bloggers, a number of us have written about the feminist potential of self-defence training. Women trained in self-defence aren't afraid to take up space, to look people in the eye, and to yell loudly if need be. Guest blogger Grace Hunt says that feminist approaches to self-defence teach us that even in a culture of sexual violence, women can act.

Feminist self-defence teaches women to take back our bodies and to find in them a source of power. Women are raised to be tiny and quiet, but the practice of martial arts cuts against that socialization. There are big movements and loud noises, and practising those movements and noises can help undo years of feminine socialization. Ann Cahill puts it this way: "So normative feminine bodily comportment not only renders women's bodies less likely to be able to respond effectively to an actual assault, but encourages women to see their own bodies as the source of the threat of assault itself. And here's my general point: this imposition of this kind of bodily comportment is harmful to all women, regardless of whether they are ever actually sexually assaulted. It limits their experience, alienates them from the full range of their bodily capacities, and pits their sense of self against their own body."[7]

Martial arts works against normative femininity, and that makes it a feminist response to living in a culture riddled with sexual violence.

When we were writing this book, a well-respected and popular radio host from CBC Radio was let go by the broadcaster because, in the CBC's words, they had learned something that made it impossible for them to continue their relationship with him.

As the story unfolded in the days following the announcement, numerous women came forward with allegations that the host had sexually assaulted and/or harassed them. For a few days, news about the firing and subsequent allegations was only thing that showed up on everyone's newsfeed.

And for the first time perhaps ever, discussions of sexual coercion and the importance of consent dominated the Canadian news. We also had a national conversation about why sexual assault goes unreported so much. We discussed it in every paper. On every television broadcast. On all the radio stations. On Facebook and Twitter, in the hallways of workplaces, and over lunch.

The national conversation drove home the extent to which it's a rare thing indeed when a woman feels confident ownership of her body—when she feels like she doesn't owe anyone anything and she gets to say "no" and let it mean "no." Not "maybe" and not "why don't you talk me into it" and not "I'm not sure" and not "maybe later," but "NO."

And when we don't feel that confident sense of ownership, it's hard not to feel insecure about choices that may upset people or make them angry or, heaven forbid, disappoint someone or not meet their expectations. Hence the level of coercion and coaxing that lots of women endure.

And so the discovery of a domain where that doesn't happen is a small miracle, like finding an oasis in the desert. And that's what jumping with both feet into an athletic activity that you love can do for you. It can make you think, "Hello! Who's been keeping this big secret from me?"

That's agency. And we could use more of it.

Is Fitness Really a Feminist Issue? You Bet!

As feminists who care about fitness, we sometimes get criticism from both sides. We hear from feminists who think fitness is trivial, a distraction from the big issues that matter. And we hear from anti-feminists who think that our feminist concern for fitness shows that all of the really important work for feminism is over and done. Because we care about fitness, both sides think we're just dusting up the crumbs after the dinner party.

But this line of thinking trivializes the very real social impact of the gendered differences in sport and fitness representation, participation, expectations, and even access and availability. Really caring for our bodies, loving our bodies, moving our bodies is a political act. Fitness isn't a trivial matter. Being able to lift and run and move heavy things around is connected to the ways we engage with the world and see ourselves as actors and agents.

We don't dispute the point that there are lots of pressing, and even lots of *more* pressing, feminist issues. Heck, we both address lots of them in our academic research, teaching, and day-to-day lives, and both of us have published widely on feminist topics other than fitness, such as transitional justice, family justice, oppression and collective responsibility, children's rights, women's agency, sexuality, and a host of other issues in feminist ethics.

We are also both engaged daily in feminist practice, organized and not organized. And we don't just mean lifting heavy weights and blogging about the ways in which fitness discourse, culture, and practice invite feminist analysis.

So we have no quarrel with the claim that feminist issues in fitness are not the only feminist issues there are. Domestic violence and violence against women more generally, lack of representation of women (let alone a diversity of women) in positions of influence and power, global poverty and its disproportionate impact on women, the restricted options available to women where employment is concerned, all sorts of issues regarding differences of privilege and oppression among and between women—all of these concerns arguably strike deeper than sport and fitness. And there are lots of other concerns about gender equality and equality more generally that warrant (and get) our attention.

Granted, then, that there are more important issues. That doesn't mean that a feminist analysis of sport and fitness is so trivial that it warrants no attention. Some of the issues we raise throughout this book call attention to significant impediments to women's flourishing: fat-shaming, body image, the tyranny of dieting, the narrow aesthetic ideal of femininity and how antithetical it is to athleticism, the sexualization of female athletes, women and competition, the way expectations about achievement are gender variable, the harms of stereotyping, issues about entitlement, inclusion, and exclusion.

What's more, we also question the very assumptions about what constitutes "fitness" in the first place. Without question we dispute the charge that there are no significant issues regarding feminism and fitness. And in many instances, sport and fitness provide us with microcosms of more general feminist concerns about power, privilege, entitlement, and socialization.

We stand firmly behind the idea that fitness is a feminist issue. Yet nowhere do we claim, nor would either of us ever claim, that fitness is the only feminist issue.

As Eve Ensler has said, "One of the most radical things women can do is to love their body. The truth of the matter is, every moment we spend worrying about our bodies, and not necessarily taking care of them, somebody is figuring out how to take money away from the poor, destroy the environment, drill, frack, burn, rape and violate women, and we're not paying attention. Be radical: Love your body!"[8] Another way of putting this idea: The less we hate and obsess about our bodies, the freer we are to change the world.

Take it away...

Feminist fitness benefits everyone, not just women. But adopting a different approach to fitness has enormous value for women. It brings confidence and empowerment into their lives, contributes to happiness, offers a solid foundation for body positivity, and even enables women as effective agents with ownership over their own lives and bodies. Fitness may not be the only feminist issue, but it's most definitely a feminist issue that warrants discussion.

Try this...

In the last "Try this..." we invited you to challenge the ways the age barrier might be holding you back. This time, try challenging gender barriers. Are you a woman who has always wanted to play baseball but didn't because that was for the boys? A man with an interest in figure skating? A genderfluid person who was slotted into gendered activities while pining for something else? Now is the time to try what you missed out on.

FOUR

The FB50 Challenge

The First Six Months—
Tracy's and Sam's Stories

September 2012 to February 2013

Tracy's Story: A Slow Start

What goes through your head when you're about to turn the page on another decade? If you're like me and so many others, you feel a strong surge of energy that challenges you to make changes—to alter the health trajectory of your future self with an intervention designed to create a more spritely version of the aging you. Marathon training, anyone? Triathlon? That aerial dance thing where you do elegant and graceful moves using long swaths of silk as props? There's something for everyone.

I started our Fittest by 50 Challenge (FB50) in September 2012, just a few weeks before my 48th birthday, as a committed yogi and walker with a history of chronic dieting and struggles with body image and body acceptance that I'm sure resonate for many women. Goals? Beyond wanting to run for 20 minutes straight by the end of 2012, I had no set goals.

Whatever I thought might happen, I had one further wish: that by my 50th birthday I would find a way to physical fitness and away from body hatred, endless dieting, weigh-ins that made me feel like crap, and joyless workouts with no purpose beyond the utilitarian aim of whipping my body into shape. Our fitness challenge wasn't just about, or even mainly about, a visible physical transformation. It offered me an opportunity to finally change my relationship with my physical self.

Two years later, by the time I turned 50, I'd completed six triathlons and was about to run a half marathon. I'd experienced (and continue to experience) a dramatic shift in how I perceive myself. I was no longer among the legions of dieters who exercise to shed weight: our two-year challenge transformed me into an athlete who trains for improved endurance, speed, and strength. With this shift, I moved into (and moved in) my body in a new way. But it took time.

September and October 2012: What the Heck Am I Doing?

My first months of the FB50 Challenge got off to a clunky beginning, with as many starts and stalls as when I learned to drive a stick shift. My sessions with a young personal trainer who equated progress with weight loss made me physically stronger, but once a week, at his behest, I had to kick off my shoes and jump on the scale in a tiny room with an ice-cold ceramic floor. Then my trainer took a tape measure to my waist, hips, thighs, and chest and jotted the numbers down in his notes. The purpose: to "track" my "progress." The thing is (and you might be familiar with this phenomenon, especially if you're a woman in mid-life), the number on the scale never budged. The measurements didn't change much either. If the scale and measurements indicate progress, what if, week in, week out, the same numbers come up on the digital read-out?

My trainer always shook his head and said, "It's probably that vegan diet. You can never get enough protein on a vegan diet.

It's almost impossible to lose weight." Really? News to me. Most everything else I'd read when I adopted my plant-based vegan diet promised that the pounds would melt away. Again, really? Not my experience. But I do it for purely ethical reasons anyway, not wanting to support the unnecessary animal suffering typical of industrialized livestock farming or the massive impact it has, proportionally, on climate change. The lesson learned: Vegan or not, some of us who want to lose weight struggle.

The FB50 Challenge prompted me to rethink my goals. Why should any of us take part in a practice that leaves us demoralized, the way weighing and measuring left me? When I told my trainer we should ditch the weekly "progress report," he winked and said, "You don't even have to look at the numbers. I'll just write them down without telling you." *Dude, do not get condescending with me. I'm old enough to be your mother.* I couldn't convince him to seek alternative ways of tracking "progress"—strength gains, increased flexibility and agility, endurance, better sleep, anything other than weight and measurements!

When I began having these conversations with my personal trainer, Sam and I had just recently started our blog, Fit Is a Feminist Issue. Through the blog, we went public about seeking a new approach to fitness that took feminism seriously. That meant taking a hard look at the way normative ideals of femininity—the slender, wispy physique of an innocent, compliant maiden—permeate popular thinking about women's physical fitness. No longer would fitness be about weight loss and becoming smaller.

But what would it look like instead? In those early days, the new picture hadn't quite come into focus for me. But I knew I wouldn't find my way if I continued to work out at a training studio that placed such a high premium on the measurements that had caused me so much suffering since my teen years.

The personal training had to stop. And before the end of the second month of the challenge, it did.

Two positives emerged from the training, however. First, it got me back to the weight room after a long hiatus. Even without the personal trainer, I had adopted weight training as an essential part of my workout week again. The second good outcome snuck up on me. My personal trainer, with his fixation on weight loss, had said, "Start running."

Back in my grad student days, I flew out of the blocks without easing into it one bit. The result: hip pain that took me out of running for the next two and a half decades. But on my trainer's advice, I pushed myself out the door. You've probably read about the incremental start—to the end of the street, around the corner, around the block. Well, it works. At first, I viewed running as a chore that I forced myself to do, like bad medicine, in small doses, three times a week, for as short a time as possible. The first time I ran 20 continuous minutes, I celebrated as if I'd just run a marathon. My friends endured many a status update on social media of my slow progress as a cautious beginner.

You may wonder about my choice to run alone instead of with others. At the time, that choice came from convenience and fear. Later, in our cardio chapter, we'll talk about the biggest perk of running: its simplicity. You throw on those shoes and head out the door. Running with others would require planning. On top of that, I had a misplaced worry that I wouldn't be able to find a slow enough group for my ability. In time, I would venture out to find a running group. But when we started the FB50 Challenge and I was flailing around trying to figure out what mattered to me, that approach scared me more than it attracted me.

I came into the challenge with yoga as the solid foundation of my activity. Every Tuesday at 6:30 a.m. my husband, Renald, and I attended an Iyengar yoga class together. We'd been going for over a decade. I feel fortunate that I'd stumbled across the Iyengar method, renowned in yoga circles for well-trained instructors who teach with precision and attend to detail. Call it the best 90 minutes I spent each week. Second best: hot yoga every Saturday and Sunday. With a rotating roster of teachers, you couldn't count on an experienced instructor, but sweating it out in a hot studio has its own special allure. Yoga, especially alongside the training

and running that I didn't yet love, showed me how much it matters that I like what I'm doing. If you've slogged it out in activities
that felt more like obligatory tasks on your to-do list than worth-
while pursuits that add joy to your life, you'll know the former as
a unique form of punishment.

I also dabbled in tai chi on my mother's encouragement. She'd
taken up this graceful, non-combative martial art in her early 70s.
Watching her work through the fluid sequence in a seamless flow
mesmerized me, so I thought, "Why not?" But I learned something about myself: to really get into a physical activity, I need it
to challenge me in a way that tai chi does not. Tai chi takes skill,
memory, grace, and agility, but I never felt exerted. Maybe when
I hit my 70s I'll go back to it, but within a few short weeks I gave
my tai chi club T-shirts to my mother and refocused my efforts on
running, yoga, and weight training.

Sam and I like to promote variety in activities. It fends off
boredom and makes it more likely that you'll find what you love.
At the same time, if you discover you don't love something, as I did
with tai chi, move on. If the very idea of having to go do a thing
fills you with dread or even just feels like a waste of precious time,
find something else.

In the first couple of months of the FB50, my attitudes about
food, dieting, and body image came into sharper view. I despise
countless features of dieting, but from my perspective, tracking
wins the "most dreaded diet practice" prize. Everyone says you
can't lose weight if you don't track your food intake: what and
how much you ate and when. Advanced trackers even record their
mood when they ate and use a hunger scale to track their hunger
levels at the beginning and at the end of a meal.

In the eighteenth century, philosopher Jeremy Bentham
designed a prison called the *panopticon*. The defining feature of
the panopticon was that prisoners couldn't tell when the guards
were watching them and when they weren't. So they self-moni-
tored, just in case. Feminist philosopher Sandra Bartky spun the
panopticon story in a uniquely feminist way. She said women

exert this kind of self-discipline over their bodies. They internalize the self-surveillance. Sound familiar? That's tracking—the panopticon in action. No thanks.

Through those early months of the FB50 Challenge, I let go of monitoring, measuring, and tracking on different levels. I stopped writing things down as much. I left my trainer because of our differences about using weight as a measure of progress. But the panopticon didn't completely go away. I shifted my focus to two new ways of keeping tabs on myself: the bod pod and sports nutrition. Guess what? Even when you're pushing 50, you can learn tough lessons. They left me feeling equally crappy.

The bod pod allegedly gives one of the most accurate body fat readings of any method available. *Maybe,* my brilliant line of thought said, *body weight is a poor measure of fitness. But what about body composition?* If you're measuring body composition, you care about the body's ratio of lean mass to fat. Ideally, you (we? I?) want a higher percentage of your body weight to be lean mass, a lower percentage to be body fat. "Getting lean," we like to call it. As a happy birthday present to myself that year, I trundled off to the bod pod, a machine at the university built for the purpose of measuring that ratio, to get an accurate reading of my body composition as a baseline for our challenge. Seriously, who inflicts this sort of punishment on herself *on her birthday?* (Spoiler: By the end of the challenge I couldn't have cared less, but we all have to start somewhere!) Ending up in the "excess fat" category, with a body fat percentage of 34.5%, made me feel about as hopeless as a bad day on the scale ever did. But, early days. I bolstered my self-esteem with that relentless optimism that reminds me so much of the beginning of any "plan." *This time it will be different.* That should have been my first clue to beware of the bod pod—if I find myself engaged in wishful thinking, trouble usually looms.

Next stop: the sports nutritionist. Leading up to the visit, she had me track my food intake for three days—because how else could she comment on what I needed to change to reach my body composition goals? Tracking, ugh. I did it anyway. She made some suggestions about vegan protein and fewer desserts and energy bars. She gave me the assurance—equally heartening and sad— that I had few changes to make. You know how it is. We don't expect to see results without huge changes, right? Thankfully, according to the sports nutritionist, my vegan diet didn't need a lot of tweaking.

It didn't stop me from setting a ridiculous body composition goal for myself. I committed to getting to 25% fat by my next birthday. That gave me a full year to work on it. How hard could it be to lose 9.5% body fat in 12 months? (Pro tip: I could more easily teleport myself to the planet Mercury.)

Here's the thing about a body composition goal: you can only get there if you focus on other things. I turned to activities. In October that year, I signed up for my very first race ever. Today, 5K is a short run for me. But that fall, I went into the 5K with Samantha, my friend Tara, and a plan to do 10:1 run-walk inter-vals (though I didn't yet know that's what they were called) for as long as it would take to complete the course. That turned out to be 36 minutes by my estimate. It was a fun race for charity, so no one got an official time. I learned that I actually did want to have a recorded time—and my running goals took shape. New goal: Get comfortable with 5K and improve my time at that distance. The fears I'd had about running and injury had drifted away.

The early months of our challenge got me reflecting on body image, too. I'm not a large woman by any stretch. I stand 5 foot 3 and at my largest I've taken a clothing size 10. For the past 10 years I've settled into the size 4 to 6 range. And yet I can still "feel fat." That fat feeling can settle in overnight, or even through the course of a day. Clothes that fit just fine when I put them on in the morning might by lunchtime start to feel like they're pinch-ing and snug, especially if I had a stressful morning. Maybe you know what I'm talking about. Even the red silk scarf, not a body-hugging item, might not look right when just yesterday it accessorized perfectly. When we feel fat, a sense of unworthiness settles in, too.

And it hardly correlates with actual body size or actual body composition. For so many women it's the go-to feeling, a stand-in for a sense of inadequacy in any area of life. This says a lot about the hold that our culture's attitudes about weight and body size has on us. Even if you attend in an explicit and conscious way to the irrational and unfair social stigma, even if you work to challenge it, you can latch onto fatness (real or imagined) as a personal deficiency. It then spirals into an energy-sucking, self-defeating stick that might make a person feel motivated to get active (but for all the wrong reasons) or leave them feeling thoroughly hopeless about exercise because it doesn't "work."

As I became aware of this dynamic within myself early in the challenge, I also discovered "feeling fit," the more positive cousin. When we feel fit, we feel strong and capable. This feeling too changes from day to day. When do you feel your fittest? If I eat ample, healthy foods—kale mix salads, quinoa bowls with tofu and rapini, or strawberries and mangoes and spinach blended into a smoothie with soy milk and pumpkin seed protein—I feel fit. These foods add high-quality fuel to my body, just what I need for the amount of activity I engage in. If I take part in things I love—yoga, running, weight training, swimming, and those wonderful seasonal treats like skiing, snowboarding, hiking, and kayaking—and I sleep enough, I own the world (or at least enough of it to make me content).

If you struggle with fat feelings, take heart. Body composition does not measure self-worth, or even fitness. And more importantly, getting a little bit active can go a long way.

November and December 2012: Time to Recalibrate

Nothing keeps a person on track through the holidays like having to blog about fitness a few times a week. Try it and you'll see for yourself. In November and December, shortly into the challenge and in the early days of the blog, I'd entrenched some good habits: yoga three to four times a week, running three times a week, resistance training three times a week in a home gym that I set up with Renald in a small space we'd set aside for yoga when we built the house eight years before.

For anyone setting up a home gym, keep it simple. Our equipment: a stability ball, a BOSU ball, two kettlebells, some dumbbells, a couple of yoga mats, and an elliptical machine that I almost never dusted off now that I'd added running. Three mornings a week Renald and I hauled ourselves out of bed in the dark and did jump squats, lunges or burpees, chest presses and military presses using the stability ball as a bench, some tricep kickbacks and bicep curls, and side lateral raises. We cycled through four different total body workout plans based on what we had learned in our months with the personal trainers.

You'll hear mixed opinions about home gyms. You've got your naysayers, who turn their noses at the limited equipment and who feel convinced that in no time at all the equipment will just become part of the furniture, taking up space but never used. On the other side, enthusiasts rhyme off all the innovative and challenging things you can do with a few dumbbells and kettlebells, combined with some body weight exercises. They believe in convenience and minimalism, and on that front it's hard to do better than we did, with the little home gym just steps away from our bed. It worked for us. We felt a strong need to prove to ourselves that we could reap all the benefits of working out with weights without having to spend thousands of dollars on personal training. That alone kept us motivated through the winter months. And having each other as workout buddies helped too.

I used the app Ease into 10K as my running guide even though, realistically, I had no plans to run 10K by the end of the winter. Not yet convinced of the value of working out with groups, I continued to run alone. I treated running as a form of meditation, and when I pictured group running, I had visions of having to push too hard to keep up with the group, falling so far behind that I'd be running alone anyway, or, worst of all, that I'd create a sense of obligation in others to slow their pace for me. Later I learned this: Some people run faster than me and some run slower. Even more surprising to me: Some people run at my pace.

By the time we hit the pre-Christmas rush, I'd lost all enthusiasm for sports nutrition counselling. Sports nutrition counselling provides solid information for the athlete who regards food as fuel for enhancing her performance—a good thing, to be sure, but if you have a history of food obsession, chronic dieting, and disordered eating, give it a pass. In my case, the diet industry had fostered in me attitudes and behaviours that cut me off from my physical hunger signals and my actual desire for food. All sense of proper portions eluded me, and still today I struggle more with how much to eat than with what to eat, whether salad or pizza, hummus and veggies or chips and salsa.

With that history, it is beyond easy for me to convince myself that a solid "plan" is not a diet. Even the diet industry avoids the word *diet* these days. But the nutrition counsellor's sound advice started me, once again, down the path of mediated eating. That's when info about what and how much I *should* eat mediates my food choices. I could feel that old obsession with food creeping back—you know, when you overthink every morsel? When you choose the salad without dressing not because that's what you want but because (supposedly) that's what makes you thin. Body acceptance went right out the window. It all started with the sports nutrition counselling. As soon as I realized what had happened, it had to go in the junk pile, right beside personal training.

January and February 2013: Off the Scale and into a New Fitness Goal

Ah, January 1st! A fresh new year invites us to write on it like a clean, blank page. With the sports nutrition approach to food behind me, performance goals more up front and centre, I returned to a way of eating that I'd first encountered almost 25 years before. In my mid-20s, I'd attempted to "recover" what I'd lost: a natural, intuitive relationship with food as a response to hunger and physical need. The most hope for a new approach came to me through the work of Geneen Roth (especially *Breaking Free from Compulsive Eating*), Jane Hirschmann and Carol

Munter (*Overcoming Overeating*), and Evelyn Tribole and Elyse Resch (*Intuitive Eating*).

Roughly, intuitive eating teaches people to reconnect with their hunger signals and stop demonizing some foods as "bad" while praising others as "good." Common to all the sources: Throw away the scale and commit to never dieting again. Sound scary? It is.

On January 1, 2013, I packed up my bathroom scale back into its original box and stuck it on a shelf so high up in my closet that I would need a stepladder to get it down. At the time of year when most people lined up for a seat in a weight loss program meeting or embarked on the latest juice "cleanse," I let go of the diet mentality. I replaced it with a more mindful way of eating.

What about activity? Sam has a talent for getting me and other unsuspecting feminist fitness types to try things just so we can blog about it. And that's how I ended up online at 10 a.m. sharp on New Year's Day, signing up for the Kincardine Women's Triathlon, a full seven and a half months in the future.

If you want to do Kincardine (which I totally recommend because, as you will see when I tell you about it later, you can't beat its awesomeness!), you need to be at the ready right at 10 or you won't get one of the precious spots. Back then, it used to fill up in a few hours. This past January 1st it sold out in less than 45 minutes. It's a great introductory triathlon—just 400 metres in Lake Huron, followed by a 12-kilometre bike ride on a mostly flat course closed to traffic and a 3-kilometre run beside the water and into a cute residential area where the neighbours cheer participants on and stand by with hoses to spray you down with cool water if you so desire. You get to experience the thrill of multi-sport, with its multiple "disciplines" and exciting transitions, but you can finish the course in a respectable time without even training because anyone in reasonable physical condition can handle the moderate distances. But as an inexperienced first-timer who had never contemplated triathlon until a few minutes before I hit "submit" on the web page to register, once the reality hit me that I'd committed to a triathlon, I might as well have signed up for an Ironman event.

Saying you're going to do a triathlon, even a teeny local triathlon like Kincardine, impresses people. At first, whenever someone said "Wow," I countered with "It's just a little triathlon." But it didn't matter. Why not? Because most people haven't even ventured into that ring at all. Triathlons of any distance have a mystique inherited from Kona, in Hawaii, where the Ironman World Championship takes place every year. People don't really care that you're not participating to such an extreme degree. Instead: *Triathlon? Wow!*

To me, it was more like: *Triathlon? Yikes!* With dieting and body weight off the table, the daunting quality of the July race gave me a whole new set of priorities. After over a decade away from the Y, I reactivated my membership so I could get back to the pool. Through the winter, I rekindled my love affair with swimming. As a first-year graduate student back in 1988, I used to go to the pool every single morning. But when I read in a magazine that swimmers hold more body fat than runners, I was shocked into replacing swimming with aerobics. I still feel sad today when I think back to how a brief paragraph in a women's fitness magazine could make me abandon an activity that kept me both physically fit and mentally grounded. When I jumped back in the pool to prepare for Kincardine, it was as if that weightless feeling of gliding through the water like a fish had never left me. I didn't yet understand what actual training should look like, but twice a week, right before lunch, I took a break from writing to do my laps at the Y.

With no strict training plan, I just added swimming to what I already had going on: running, yoga, and weight training. Nothing systematic went into my decision about frequency. Once a week struck me as inadequate for anything. So I scheduled each activity at least twice, three times for running and weights. Peering into the murky future, I could see that my calendar might get overcrowded once spring came and I added cycling to the mix.

But like many a newbie, I fumbled my way through the first few months of triathlon training, forging ahead on my own, without guidance. Do I recommend that way of going about it? Um ... no. If you're going to do triathlon, you can join a club or talk to a coach or sign up for a beginners' program at your local Y or community centre. You can even go online and find training plans, tips, and strategies for getting started and for training. Options abound. Of course, I took none of them that winter.

But I'm all for taking a forgiving attitude toward new activities and seeing where that takes me. I had something to get excited about and, for the first time in my life, a goal race. Training for a specific event, not to drop pounds or look a certain way, had an appealing novelty to it.

And I liked it.

TRACY'S TYPICAL TRAINING WEEK, SEPTEMBER 2012–FEBRUARY 2013

MONDAY	7 A.M. WEIGHT TRAINING
TUESDAY	6:30 A.M. YOGA AT THE IYENGAR STUDIO; 10 A.M. TAI CHI (SEPTEMBER–OCTOBER)/ SWIMMING (JANUARY–FEBRUARY)
WEDNESDAY	7 A.M. WEIGHT TRAINING; 11 A.M. RUN BEFORE LUNCH
THURSDAY	10 A.M. TAI CHI (SEPTEMBER–OCTOBER)/ SWIMMING (JANUARY–FEBRUARY)
FRIDAY	7 A.M. WEIGHT TRAINING AND A SHORT RUN
SATURDAY	8:30 A.M. HOT YOGA
SUNDAY	8:30 A.M. HOT YOGA; 2 P.M. RUN

What's wrong with that picture? No rest days—I'll talk about my rest day "issues" later. And we have a good section on the importance of rest and recovery in our chapter about keeping it realistic.

Sam's Story: The Adult Onset Athlete

The Fittest by 50 Challenge story isn't for either of us about inactive, out-of-shape people discovering exercise for the very first time. For each of us, it was a matter of upping our game to get ready for the years ahead. I wanted to start the second half of life (as some people ambitiously say) at my peak so I could keep moving and doing the things I love. Looking around my department at work, I began to see a pretty big range in what a person's 50s, 60s, and 70s might look like, and who fell into what end of the spectrum seemed to partially turn on staying fit. As we age, it seems, the gap between those who stay active and those who don't gets bigger and doors start to close. I wanted to keep doors open as long as I could.

I love physical activity and think of it as part of the fun side of life. It's not a duty—it's recreation. I grew up swimming and riding my bike, and although I never played sports, I loved to run and jump about, like most kids. Later, with my partner, Jeff, I rode bikes, played a variety of sports, and generally shared an active outdoorsy lifestyle. When we had children of our own, I was happy to share our pursuits with them. For vacations we camped and canoed and cross-country skied and biked. While the kids took swimming classes at the local YMCA, I worked out lifting weights and took spin classes in the studios upstairs. Now I have teen athletes in the house and we have a pretty active life together. My daughter and I do martial arts. One son lifts weights and runs with me. My other son is the family champion for long nature hikes and keeps trying to lure me into rock climbing.

But of all the things I do, it's riding my bike I love the most. My love of bike riding started as a kid but took a brief hiatus in high school. I think I was too cool, too busy, and too bookish to even consider doing anything active then. It wasn't until university, in Halifax, when a friend riding her bike across Canada from the west coast abandoned her bike with me—deciding instead to take the bus and ferry to Newfoundland—that I got attached to cycling as an adult. I remember riding her bike that summer and then, the week before she was due home, taking it into a bike shop, and asking them for one of my own. It turns out, no surprise, I couldn't afford one like hers, so I settled on an entry-level hybrid city bike and charged it to my very first credit card.

My love of lifting weights began a few years later, in graduate school, when I decided that if I was going to be big, I was also going to be strong. I'm not that tall—just 5 foot 7—but I'm pretty solidly built. I put on muscle easily. Model thinness just isn't a possibility for me, given the body I've got.

Grad students got a tuition waiver, which meant no fees for classes, including undergraduate physical education courses. I passed on riflery and golf, but I did sign up for Introduction to Sailing (my husband raced sailboats and we wanted to do some double-handed races together) and for Fundamentals of Weight Training. In that class I learned to bench press, squat, and deadlift for university credit. Sadly, I only got a B and I had to explain my transcript to potential employers—that the course listed on the transcript just as "Fundamentals" wasn't a philosophy class at all.

My adult weight has ranged between 155 and 235 pounds, though I'm not sure the lowest number counts. I might have stayed there just for a day! I've done the complete cycle, up and down and up again, a couple of times at least. I weighed the lowest number at my wedding and then never again. But I was at my absolute thinnest in high school, and also, then, my least fit. I smoked and drank black coffee, looked great, but couldn't walk a flight of stairs without getting out of breath. Unlike other women, I've never had aspirations of being slim. It's not my body type. At my lightest, my BMI (body mass index) still read as "overweight."

While I began the challenge with a history of cycling and weightlifting, it was only in my mid-life that my self-conception as an athlete took hold. I jokingly call myself an "adult onset athlete." As I approached 40, I began running, tried a triathlon, and bought a road bike. Since then I've been doing long rides, riding with bike clubs, racing a bit here and there. On most of my holidays, my bike comes along for the ride.

I've always been an active person, so why the FB50 Challenge? Fifty seemed to scream out for something new and for something positive. As I looked at the decades ahead, it was clear to me that I wanted them to be full of activity. I wanted to start mid-life at my fittest. For me, fitness is a launching pad that makes new adventures possible. My goal was to be able to try new things—rock climbing, mountain biking, trail running—without worrying about a fitness barrier. It's great to be able to focus on skills without worrying about being out of breath.

While Tracy and I debated what counts as "fitness," it was clear that, for me, versatility mattered. There's no one big fitness goal for me. And so my FB50 Challenge focused on trying new things—rowing and CrossFit—and adding distance on my bike. I also successfully tested for a new belt level in Aikido, a Japanese martial art that I do. The month before my 50th birthday I rode my bike from Toronto to Montreal, about 600 kilometres in total, much of it along the beautiful Great Lakes Waterfront Trail, as part of the Friends for Life Bike Rally in support of people living with HIV/AIDS.

During our challenge I also branched out in my approach to nutrition. I engaged a sports nutritionist, tried using that same fancy machine Tracy talked about—the bod pod—to measure my body fat percentage, and did a year-long program of online nutrition counselling. I've long had a hatred of diets and restrictive ways of eating, but I wanted to learn more about nutrition and about the connection between eating well and performing well physically. It's not that I wouldn't love to lose weight, but in the end I'm more interested in health than in thinness, and in sports performance over performance at a weekly weigh-in. I'm active and happy the size I am now, although I struggle a bit with terminology. Others might call me "fat," but I don't see myself that way. I'm pretty muscular and strong, and I think of myself as "big" more than "fat."

When the FB50 Challenge began, I was still often wondering about goals and ambitions. Who's the fittest version of me? What specific goals do I want to set for myself? I'm an adult onset athlete, that's true, but I've had other periods of my life where I've gotten serious about one thing or another. In graduate school it was weightlifting. In my late 30s, it was running, when I ran off 60 pounds—and acquired two stress fractures as a result. Later, in my mid-40s, it was cycling, both track and road, with some short distance triathlons and duathlons thrown in for good measure.

This time around I was looking forward, to 50 and to well past 50. I wanted to enter middle age with a strong, versatile fitness base. I wanted to be both strong and fast. I wanted to try lots of different things. Friends have always joked that I'm an attention deficit disorder exerciser. I like to do a variety of sports and physical activities. I wanted a future where I could stay active and in which when I tried a new thing, I could focus on skills, not whether I was fit enough.

My main sport going into the FB50 Challenge was going to remain cycling, mostly road. During the challenge, I said, I was going to try to keep running out of it. There was lots else I liked to do. Why bother with something that hurts? I also enjoyed throwing large men around while wearing white robes as a serious student of Aikido. It's a beautiful martial art, really, but at the time I was struggling with it. I was also lifting weights. When the challenge began, I'd just started CrossFit, which I was loving for its high-intensity, high-energy workouts. CrossFit is a popular gym program that includes elements from high-intensity interval training, Olympic weightlifting, plyometrics, powerlifting, and gymnastics. I was also playing soccer and, when I wanted to stretch, taking hot yoga.

I began the challenge as an above-average-size person who struggled with our society's expectation that all athletes look like fitness models and that fat women aren't active. I wanted to lose weight, mostly to make it up hills faster and to avoid injury, but wasn't prepared to sacrifice performance in either the strength or speed department to do it. I was also worried about how realistic weight loss was as a goal, given the stats on dieting and success. For the most part, I knew, I wanted to focus on fitness.

So what were my specific goals going into this challenge?

I had a few. I knew wanted to get faster on the bike and to take my road cycling more seriously. I wanted to improve my power to weight ratio, which matters a lot for cyclists. That means getting stronger and lighter. And I wanted to try something new. I wanted to start my 50s in peak fitness to offset the tendency to slow down as we age. But overall, my fitness focus was on having fun and trying new things.

Who Likes Sports Nutrition and Tracking? I Do, I Do!

I began the challenge committed to the idea that, for me, this wasn't about weight loss. Been there, done that, a couple of times. But like many busy women, with a big job and a house full of teenagers, my own nutrition often took a back seat. I was interested in revamping my eating with sports nutrition rather than in weight loss as a goal. In the first six months of our challenge, I met with a sports nutritionist and tried to shape up my nutrition for performance goals.

I went into the meeting with Jennifer the nutritionist with my food logs for the weeks past all filled out. I'm a natural tracker even when I'm not eating that well. Tracy asks, Who likes tracking? I do! I plan meals, I count grams of protein, and I track. Mostly it feels liberating. Sometimes it feels like a chore. But in a hectic family with lots of meals, snacks, and groceries on the go, my food log often serves as a way to remind me that what I eat matters. For me, it's much more about making sure I take care of myself than it is a reminder to eat less. The changes Jennifer recommended weren't big ones, really. I vowed to start keeping healthy snacks at work to avoid arriving home ravenous.

What's in a Label? Fit and Fat/Big/Brawny

I began the challenge with an ambivalent relationship with the label "fat." I do often claim to be "fit and fat," but I'm never quite sure if *fat* is the word I want. When I was writing on the blog, I'd sometimes claim that word, but it doesn't really fit me. This isn't because the word *fat* makes me ashamed. I'm all about reclaiming labels, and I'm a tremendous fan of the Health at Every Size movement. I also recognize that according to the numbers on the scale and my BMI, I'm significantly overweight. And I know that some people see me as fat. Others don't, though. I'm most likely to claim the label when some well-meaning person within earshot starts equating being fat with being out of shape—thinking what exactly, that I'll agree with them? Sometimes they say, "Oh, we don't mean *you*. You're not fat, really." Then I want to remind people that I'm part of the story too. When we start talking about the statistics, I want in.

So why the ambivalence? I began the challenge wearing size 12 or size 14—well within the range of easily available sizes—and I don't feel particularly fat. The bits of me that have clothes issues relate to muscles and women's clothing styles: biceps, shoulders, and calves. So I sometimes use the label "fat," but I often feel squeamish about it, as if I don't really belong in the club.

What's the alternative? At Aikido I started to notice the vocabulary we have to describe male bodies. We often joke about how much fun it is to throw the "big" guys. Someone commented that I should pay attention to how they roll because they have to do it with more finesse to avoid crashing into the mats. (A mistake I make from time to time. Ouch, sore shoulder!) And the big men are big in different ways. Some are overweight; others are tall; some are extremely muscular, such as the powerlifter in the club. But there's no angst in referring to them as "big."

We have other positive words too. My favourite is *brawny*. No need for further explanation or apology. Brawny men are fun to throw. I'd much rather play Aikido with one of them than with a frail person I'd worry about hurting. Their large bodies feel resilient and strong. Why can't we feel the same way about big women?

And please don't get me started on all the cutesy labels women use to avoid the word *fat*: "fluffy," "chunky," "chubby"...

So I began the challenge as "fat," I guess. But "big" suits me better. And I knew that no matter what, given my muscles and build, I'd *always* be big.

With a little nutrition advice in hand, my thought for the first six months was to try to lose some fat and gain, or at least keep, muscle while doing so. Like Tracy, I had a visit with a clinic on campus that measures your body fat percentage using a machine called the bod pod. Basically you sit in it in a bathing suit and find out what portion of your weight is composed of fat—your lean mass to fat ratio. I confirmed that the standard weight recommendations are probably too low for me given that I was more than 130 pounds of bone and muscle. It helped to know that, and to be realistic about what's possible for me in terms of losing weight and staying strong. I was able to stay focused on nutrition and strength throughout the challenge, and this was a good place to begin.

Row, Row, Row the Boat: Trying Something New

One of the reasons I love being fit is the ability to try new things and be able to focus on skills rather than basic fitness. I learned to compete in cross country, as a runner, for just that reason. Soon after my 48th birthday I got an email from a friend of a friend who'd just moved to London. Her partner was a serious rower and wanted to start coaching a women's rowing group. Did I want in?

Yes, yes, yes. Pick me! Pick me!

I've always wanted to try rowing, and rowing has always been a big deal here in London, Ontario. I'd often admired rowers—rowing looks so beautiful, and like cyclists, rowers get to play outside in the sunrise. I loved watching people at rowing practice as I rode alongside on the bike paths. But it's nothing I'd ever done before.

I had been tempted in the past to try rowing but had been put off by weight categories. Lightweight rowers are tiny. I think the cut-off might be 130 pounds for women, but the heavyweights tend to Amazon proportions. Often they're 6 feet tall or more. When I was younger I would have been strongly encouraged to "make weight" to row as a lightweight, I think. I'm only 5 foot 7 and in theory it would be doable, but not, these days, without ditching some muscle. That matters less, however, for a masters-level rower and when competing for fun. At the encouragement of a friend, I started attending indoor training sessions at the London Rowing Club and I joined their Off-Water Masters Program as a beginner. Since it was Canada, in the autumn and winter we would be training inside for quite a few months, though they also had a tank for practising in-water technique.

Our first coached day covered basic erg technique. *Erg* is short for *ergometer,* the name for a rowing machine that measures how much you are working.

The second day of indoor training was our first two-kilometre erg test. Here I discovered that rowers and cyclists have something in common: a love of suffering! So that was one transferable skill from cycling.

Since I have no shame and since part of the joy of a new sport is that I have no idea how bad I'm doing, I was happy to share my results on our blog. I was a beginner again, and I loved that. We repeated these erg tests monthly and results were posted on the bulletin board at the club so we could track progress. I'm just a little bit competitive (even if only with myself), so I liked that.

In November I did my first 2K time trial. Rowers regularly do a 2K time trial to test their progress. That's why you'll notice a preset 2K program on the ergs in your gym. A split is a timed segment, and in the 2K time trial there are five 400-metre splits. For my first time trial, I had a total time of 8:45.4 and an average split time of 2:11.4. Those numbers established the base from which I was starting.

What I really liked about indoor rowing in those first six months was that we had a keen coach. I needed that. And I liked that we had to push ourselves to the limit, which fits my sports profile. A time trial is a time trial. There was a great group of women, mostly around my age. I also took part in a local ergatta and won!

An ergatta, like a rowing regatta but indoors, uses rowing machines. That fall I competed in a very nice, locally organized event for high schoolers, the London High School Invitational Ergatta, to which we'd added a masters class event. It was just our local group racing, at our home club, which also made it less nerve-racking.

I enjoyed the mood and the atmosphere: the young racers, keen coaches, and excited parents. It was fun to watch their technique and see some of the blazing fast times of the seniors just finishing high school, on their way to university rowing teams. Our masters group arrived early and we had ample time to warm up with the ergs set aside in the space we usually use as a kitchen and meeting room.

Our coach gave us some terrific advice in the days leading up to the race. He told us to pick a 500-metre split time for which we'd aim in advance. Don't try to wing it. "Pick something that you think will be challenging, but—importantly—something you're confident you can hit." His advice was to settle into that split time as soon as possible, ignore the adrenaline rush from the start (which was very hard for me—I'm a go out fast and collapse kind of gal!), and save our energy for the final sprint. He said, two kilometres is longer than you think. And yes, indeed, it is. You can't all-out sprint for eight minutes, but eight minutes isn't quite an endurance event either. Two kilometres is a tough distance. He advised us to wait till the last 250 metres and then take up the pace, going all out with everything we had left for the final 50 to 100 metres.

And it worked!

My 500-metre split times went down in the monthly two-kilometre tests we'd been doing, from 2:11 for the very first one to 2:07. I picked 2:07 as the pace I'd maintain, and while I couldn't quite resist the urge to sprint a bit off the start, I did remember the coach's advice and held it steady at 2:07 for a long stretch.

I had lots left in the tank to sprint at the end, finishing with a 2:04 split time—a new personal best.

I also won the women's masters category, and finished first after the guys. I won a new hat. But really, the new personal best mattered more, since I knew there were women who would have beat me if they'd raced. Winning in a time trial like that is partly a matter of luck: it's who shows up.

Also, for some people it was their first time racing. It was my first rowing race but not my first race. I've done lots of running, triathlon, and bike races. And knowing how to handle getting ready for a race and how to deal with pre-race jitters helped, I think.

In this first race I finished with a total time of 8:16. My new goal was for a sub-eight-minute time, which seemed doable if I were to stick with rowing throughout the challenge.

That fall was a great introduction to rowing, and I loved learning something new. The sport turned out to be very technical, and after a season of indoor training, I'd never be able to look at people using the rowing machines at the gym the same way again.

Women and Men in White Pajamas: I ♥ Aikido

I love Aikido. I really do. But I struggled during the first six months of the challenge with whether Aikido loved me back enough for me to continue. At times it felt like a classic bad romance. In the fall I was entering my sixth year of training at the Aiki Budo Centre (ABC) of London, with two years off during sabbaticals in Australia and New Zealand, where I dabbled with other forms of Aikido. I recommend Aikido to all of my friends who want to try a martial art. I was also training with my daughter at the Western Aikido Club on the university campus. (Both ABC and WAC practise the Yoshikan style of Aikido. It's a more martial, less flowy version of this martial art.)

I started Aikido when my kids were younger. It was the one activity that had attracted both sons—the ballet dancer and the now football and rugby player. One liked its grace and beauty, and the other liked the more martial aspects. That is, he liked the fighting! After about six months of watching the boys and thinking it looked fun, I noticed that some of the parents stuck around for the adult class and the children stayed in the room and played. Now it's my 20-year-old daughter and me who are students of Aikido. Her brothers have moved on, as teenagers do, but I hope one day they'll come back.

I love lots of things about Aikido. First, the structure, the rhythm, and the ritual of Aikido are beautiful. I love bowing in and feeling like we are creating a special, sacred place. We create the mood of seriousness and mindful playfulness.

And where else do you get to learn how to fall? I keep thinking that senior citizens should all take Aikido just for the practice in falling. A few winters ago I hit the ice getting out of my car and went for a wild ride. I had never been sure if the techniques I'd learned in Aikido would be useful, but I didn't even think. I just rolled properly and didn't hurt a thing, pride aside. It was so nice to know that after all that practice, my Aikido falling technique had become second nature. And while I'm not usually that taken with the psychological and spiritual aspects of martial arts, there really is something about being knocked down and getting back up again hundreds and hundreds of times that's very useful in life.

I also love that Aikido is such a gentle martial art. It's a self-defence technique that works by redirecting the energy of one's attacker. When Aikido is done right, the movement of one's partner is not forceful, but it can't be resisted (well, not without a great deal of unnecessary pain). I'm not convinced I'd execute any of our techniques perfectly if I were attacked, but I'm certain I don't look like an easy target. I know how to walk with confidence. I can yell pretty loudly in someone's face, and I am pretty sure I'd be able to strike someone and knock them to the ground if need be.

The diversity of the participants is another welcome and refreshing feature of Aikido. Aikido is the activity I do with the greatest range of age, size, backgrounds of other practitioners. I really enjoy my Aikido companions—a welcome switch from university life ... We get to know each other's bodies well. I can tell you who has the flexible shoulders, who has stiff knee joints, and who bounces really well when thrown. We lend our bodies to one another to train, and that takes a lot of trust. I need to know that if I tap on the mat, my training partner will stop applying the technique they're using on me. It's a pretty special community.

Our teachers are volunteers and they're wonderful. They give so much to the community and are excellent both as teachers of technique and as role models. There's terrific leadership and a real sense that they work as a team.

And of course, as I mentioned before, I like throwing big men around the dojo. It's satisfying to know you've got a technique right because you can fling someone much stronger and larger around the room. They also make good noises when they land. "Whee! Thump!" we joke, though our goal is less thumping and more quiet, soft landings.

But I also struggle with some of what confronts me in Aikido. Like rolling! I'm lousy at rolling, and sometimes I hurt myself. I keep trying but it's not coming easily. Then there's the kneeling. It's not the most comfortable position for everyone, and it really hurts my knees.

Also, I wonder sometimes where the women are. I wish there were more women on the mats. There are some, but only a couple of the black belts are women. In that respect it reminds me of the university, where women make up such a small percentage of the highest ranks.

Learning how to hit people was a huge challenge that I have to work at. If I don't put enough energy into a technique, my training partner can't learn how to defend himself. If my punch stops a few inches shy of my partner's face, he isn't really learning to block.

And then there are some of the mental challenges, like learning the names of techniques in Japanese and trying not to stress too much about testing. Testing makes me nervous, though I'm getting better about that. I don't like people watching me, but once I'm in the zone and concentrating on the technique, I forget that people are there.

One of my goals starting out the challenge was to test for a new belt in Aikido. It's not one of those martial arts in which progression is guaranteed, a normal matter of course. Some people, like me, train for years, at a middle rank. In the end I tested for two belts during our FB50 Challenge, but I struggled a lot during the first six months with whether or not to stick with it.

In favour of sticking with it, despite my struggles with rolling and my discomfort with testing, was that sometimes you learn the most when things aren't easy. For athletically talented people, some sports play on our strengths and others don't. Often we are best at the ones we come to with a great deal of natural talent and then build from there.

In favour of moving on, I sometimes thought—with my philosopher's hat on—about how there are dozens (probably hundreds, maybe even thousands) of motivational posters praising hard work, perseverance, and determination, but very few sing the praises of cutting your losses and moving on. Sometimes it makes sense to quit, and Aikido was hard. Aristotle describes a virtue as a "mean" or "intermediate" between two extremes: the extreme of excess and the extreme of deficiency. Most people quit things too easily. Exercise plans, French classes, and piano lessons spring immediately to mind. And successful people, we're told, stick to it—they have determination. I suspect, given that most people go wrong in this direction, that determination makes sense as the virtue to encourage.

But people can also go wrong in the other direction, sticking with something long past the point where sticking with it makes sense. People stay in bad jobs and bad relationships, counting the time put in (sunk costs) for far more than it's worth. Successful people also know when to quit. It turns out that trying lots of things, cutting your losses early, and moving on is a trait many high achievers share.

I seriously considered quitting Aikido when it appeared that I had trained and trained and trained and I wasn't being invited to test. My progress was too slow (glacial, even), there were lots of other physical activities I was good at, and I'm the sort of person who needs progress. I also worried that I hurt myself too much and that Aikido endangered other physical activities I was loathe to give up. At the higher belt levels, people seem to do only Aikido (not Aikido and other sports), and I'm all about well-roundedness. Aikido is also an indoor activity, and for the most part I much preferred being outside.

In the end, I decided to take the bad news about not testing stoically, work hard, continue to train as if I was going to test (a great way to polish up the techniques), and reassess come spring when the call of the outdoors was a little louder. And weirdly, good news came out of relaxing about it all. I went ahead and trained extra hard without thinking about the test, and with the help of some very special people, I was invited to test in Aikido after all. I was loud and I was confident and I started to feel good about Aikido again.

SAM'S TYPICAL TRAINING WEEK, SEPTEMBER 2012–FEBRUARY 2013

MONDAY	**REST DAY! (BUT I STILL COMMUTE BY BIKE AND WALK THE DOG.)**
TUESDAY	**6–7 A.M. CROSSFIT; AFTERNOON INDOOR ROWING; 7–8 P.M. OPEN CLASS, AIKIDO**
WEDNESDAY	**5 P.M. BIKE RIDE, 40 KM, WEATHER AND DAYLIGHT DEPENDING**
THURSDAY	**6–7 A.M. CROSSFIT; AFTERNOON INDOOR ROWING; 7–8:30 P.M. AIKIDO ADVANCED CLASS**
FRIDAY	**7–8 A.M. CROSSFIT**
SATURDAY	**10–11 A.M. AIKIDO**
SUNDAY	**12–4 P.M. LONG BIKE RIDE—60–100 KM (UNTIL THE FALL, AND THEN MORE INDOOR ROWING); 8 P.M. SOCCER GAME**

PART TWO

MOTIVATION: Why Get Fit?

FIVE

Sure, Let's Get Fit, but Fit for What?

PHILOSOPHERS REVEL in asking and answering questions. There's even a joke about it: *How many philosophers does it take to change a lightbulb? It depends on what you mean by "change."* So, we're both philosophers, and it's no surprise that when Sam started the "What would it mean to be the fittest we've ever been by the time we turn 50?" conversation on Facebook, we couldn't easily land on one measure. We had our own thoughts about what was important to us personally, but anyone taking on such a challenge needs to decide on their own. What does it mean to be the "fittest"? Is it about speed? Strength? Endurance? Flexibility? Is it about body weight? Body composition? What about attitude? Health, yes, but does that include mental and spiritual health?

Let's have a closer look at the various options.

Zoom, Zoom: Is Faster Fitter?

One easy way to measure fitness is speed at a particular activity. Most runners can tell you their best 5K or 10K times. High school cross-country runners regularly test their mile time, and track runners their 100 and 400 metre times. As a cyclist, Sam regularly tracked her time trial speeds and times across the season, looking for an easy measure of improvement with training. When she trained regularly with a bike team, they used to do two 5K time trials (with a short rest in between) each month after a rest or low-volume training week, to test if they'd adequately recovered. Riders who spend time in the velodrome come to know their 500 metre, 1 kilometre, and 3 kilometre times. During Sam's foray into rowing she did monthly 2 kilometre erg tests to track fitness. Speed tracks progress.

Speed is a great regular check-in when you've got one sport and you're tracking your progress over time. But if you're like us and involved in multiple different sports, it's a challenge. *Which* sport? What times? Sam knew her past running times, but when she started the FB50 Challenge, injuries held her running in check. As a new runner, Tracy had no old times to use as benchmarks. Neither of us is particularly speedy, and we also wanted and needed a broader fitness focus than just speed. So while we would use speed measures in our training, they wouldn't become our primary focus. But for someone else, someone more focused on one sport, speed might be a good measure of progress and make perfect sense.

Stronger, Fitter?

Strength is another important element of fitness. Think about the typical person's day at the gym. Most workouts include both cardio and strength training. And with good reason. Even committed runners, for example, care also about developing strength to prevent injury and aid recovery.

Not long ago, women were discouraged from strength training. People feared that if women lifted weights, they would "bulk up" and start to look like men (gasp!). Instead the amorphous "they" of popular media encouraged women to "tone" and use light weights with high repetitions. Besides the association of muscularity with masculinity, this message did women a serious disservice.

For the woman who isn't focused on one particular sport, strength really matters, especially as we age. Women who lift weights have better bone strength and can stave off the loss of muscle that comes with aging. Indeed, recent research has shown that you can start strength training and see real benefits at any age. One 12-month study conducted at Tufts University showed that with just two days a week of progressive strength training, postmenopausal women hip and spine bone density increased by 1%, their strength by 75%, and their dynamic balance by 13%, while the control group *lost* bone, strength, and balance.[1] Strength training also reduces risk for falls and fractures. The societal pressure on women to stay away from the weight room isn't a trivial matter. This kind of everyday sexism exerts a real cost on women's well-being.

Things are different for young women though, right? After all, isn't "strong the new skinny"? In the changing trends in women's body shapes and sizes, muscular is in. At least a certain kind of muscularity: visible abs, low body fat percentage, chiselled shoulders, and arms like Michelle Obama's. "Strong" in this sense is a look rather than an achievement that comes from training. The women athletes who compete in the CrossFit games have that "look." What we don't see is all the other women, of all different shapes and sizes, who do CrossFit. Fitness ought to be about athletics, not aesthetics. Let's celebrate the top women in CrossFit for their speed and strength, not how they look.

Strength does have one big advantage: it's easy to measure. Powerlifters have a set series of lifts that they track (bench, deadlift, and squat), and so do Olympic lifters (the snatch and the clean and jerk). Recently, with the rise of CrossFit, there's been a return to bodyweight lifts such as the pull-up and the muscleup. Both of us care about strength. We've tracked and measured our progress across various lifts. Despite not using strength as a single measure, each of us had strength training as an essential part of our FB50 Challenge, and we recommend it for everyone.

She Who Endures: Endurance and Cardiovascular Fitness

Back in the '80s we called it "aerobics" or "aerobic fitness." Think Lycra, slouchy knit leg warmers, and Jane Fonda. Today, you're more likely to hear people talking about "cardio" and "cardiovascular fitness." Most fitness plans have a cardio component, designed to improve our fitness on this measure.

What is cardiovascular health? It's a measure of the body's ability to take in, transport, and use oxygen during exercise. When your cardiovascular health improves, it means that your lungs are taking in lots of oxygen and your heart is pumping that oxygen through the bloodstream, delivering it to working muscles better than it used to. Those muscles, in turn, use that oxygen more efficiently.

We sometimes forget that the heart is a muscle. As all muscles do, the heart gets stronger when it works. Adding a cardio component to your workout helps to strengthen that muscle. To get the heart pumping harder and faster, we can try walking, running, swimming, cycling, stair climbing, cross-country skiing, or even one of those familiar aerobics classes with snappy music and an enthusiastic instructor bellowing out commands.

The most accurate metric for cardiovascular fitness is VO_2 max. That's the maximum amount of oxygen your body can use during exercise at maximum effort: the millilitres of oxygen used in one minute per kilogram of body weight. That number goes up when your aerobic fitness improves. VO_2 max can be tested in a number of different ways, all of which involve going "all out" (maximum effort!) for longer than feels comfortable, sometimes until you can't continue. An excellent VO_2 max for women aged 40 to 60 is in the 36 to 48 range. Elite endurance athletes have extremely high VO_2 max scores, which means their bodies use oxygen more efficiently than the rest of us. For example, cross-country skier

Bjørn Dæhlie has an extraordinary VO_2 max of 90. Marathon runner Joan Benoit's VO_2 max is 78.6, in the same range as many elite endurance runners. VO_2 max is a good indicator of aerobic endurance.

Genetics matter, but you can improve your VO_2 max through training. If you're committed to endurance sports, as Tracy is, then you'll want to do things that increase your VO_2 max. To do that, you need to do some high-intensity interval training (HIIT), adding some blasts of near maximum effort to any aerobic training.

We'll talk more about HIIT in the chapter on cardio and cross-training. But for now let's just say this: back in the day, we mid-lifers didn't do intensity. Everyone told us to aim for at or just below our "aerobic heart rate" to achieve "maximum fat burning." Allegedly, we could establish thresholds based roughly on our maximum heart rate, the calculation for women being 220 minus your age (for example, if you're 50, then your maximum heart rate is 170 beats per minute). Different percentages of the maximum constituted different zones. The 50–65% range was deemed the "fat-burning zone," and 65–80% was good for both aerobic conditioning and fat burning. Using the example again of an average 50-year-old based on the rough calculation, working out in that zone would put them somewhere around 85 to 100 beats per minute.

But if you've got any amount of fitness at all, just the thought of a long session in the fat-burning zone leaves you cold. Tracy, nowhere near an elite athlete, wouldn't even break a sweat if she had to work out at a heart rate between 85 and 100 beats per minute. But she used to do it. One summer she read all of *War and Peace* on a stationary bike at the Y. If her heart rate ever went over the fat-burning zone, it was only because of a high-drama scene in the book! Endurance and cardio training are important for overall fitness. To get results in training, you'll want to up the intensity. If you do that, your VO_2 max will increase. That translates into the ability to push yourself harder for longer.

Get Bent: Flexibility as a Measure of Fitness

Can you touch your toes with your legs straight? Sit in the full lotus position in a yoga class? Were you the kid who could easily move into a backbend in gym class? Or did you envy that kid?

Flexible people have lots of range of movement in their joints. And flexibility is an important element of overall physical health. You would do well to work on it, because the things we do for strength and cardio health can actually *decrease* range of motion.

Most well-rounded fitness programs include stretching as part of the warm-up or cool-down. As we age, we reach a time when we need longer arms if we want to touch our toes without bending our knees. Good news: By focusing on flexibility, we can keep working with the arms we have!

Yoga, when done properly—with attention to alignment and props to help when tight joints make a pose unavailable—can help make us more flexible. With regular practice, most people see change, even if that change shows up in tiny increments. Tracy once did a workshop with a teacher in her 70s who, when she turned 50, set herself this goal: to be able to do full lotus by the time she turned *80*. So yes, it's a process for everyone. And it's well worth the long-term effort. More flexibility can mean less lower back pain, since tight hamstrings are often the culprit for people with chronic issues in their lower backs.

Flexibility alone is not a marker of good health, though. In yoga classes, experienced instructors sometimes talk about the dangers of being "naturally flexible." Tracy's teacher speaks of the difference between "holding" a pose, with the muscles are actively engaged around the joints and bones, and "hanging out" in a pose. When we just "hang out," we're passive in a way that could damage or overdo the stretch instead of working into it. If you're like Tracy and have a tendency to hyperextend, that is, to move joints like knees and elbows beyond their natural range, any good yoga teacher will teach you to hold back in certain poses or even to use bolsters or blocks for support, to act as "brakes" and prevent injury.

And besides needing to be cautious about overstretching or hyperextending, we've all known people who can bend and twist but who don't take care of themselves in other ways. Someone might do really well in a 90-minute yoga class but struggle to carry heavy bags of groceries. Even though flexibility isn't a stand-alone benchmark for fitness, it's a great thing to work on. And if you're already flexible, it's a good idea to complement that natural gift with strength training.

Finding Your Equilibrium: Balance and Coordination

Another benefit often associated with yoga, but also found in tai chi, martial arts, and even cardio classes that sometimes include complex movements, is improved balance and coordination. Can you do the yoga pose known as "tree"? To do that you need to stand on one leg and bend the other out to the side so that the foot rests on your thigh, then you either bring your hands together in front of your chest in prayer position or extend your arms high above your head. It's a tricky pose that requires balance as you try to stay steady in one place. Balance requires strength and stability.

Coordination is sometimes defined as "the ability to use different parts of the body together smoothly and efficiently." Any complex activity, such as riding a bike, swimming, skating, or even walking, requires coordination. When we first start out with a new activity, we often feel awkward and, quite literally, uncoordinated. Think back to your first dance lesson, first time on skis, first attempt at tennis, or first time throwing a javelin (haven't thrown a javelin yet? Give it a try!). Much of the frustration of being a novice is lack of coordination. Coordination is an important aspect of success in most physical activities and sports.

Together, balance and coordination are foundational. We need a basic sense of balance and coordination in order to get started. But these can also improve. Think again to riding a bike, which requires both balance and coordination. Tracy relived that all over again when she switched to clipless pedals (the kind that require you to snap your shoe cleats into your pedals). Suddenly, with the added element of being attached to her pedals and unable to put her foot down, it threw off her balance and coordination. But she did eventually experience that sense of achievement when balance and coordination came together while clipped in. Samantha regularly challenges her balance and timing with the practice of Aikido. Aikido techniques rely on having a strong, stable stance and on responding to a strike in a way that takes your opponent, or training partner, off balance while you remain strong and stable.

While not the only markers or measures of fitness, both balance and coordination are significant indicators that you're making positive gains.

The Biggest Loser: Body Weight as a Measure of Fitness

When many women set out on a program of fitness, they begin by stepping on the scale. What's easier to measure than weight? People draw such a strong association between fitness and thinness that the vast majority find it hard to believe that fat people can be fit or that thin people can be out of shape.

You might be thinking, okay, maybe not weight but BMI (body mass index) matters. But just two variables, weight and height, determine BMI. We think of BMI as weight dressed up for Sunday dinner. Researchers never intended BMI to be used to assess the health of individuals. They developed it as a way of looking at size across populations. BMI also fails to distinguish between fat and lean mass. Many Olympic athletes and almost all professional football players count as overweight or obese using BMI as a measure.

We both know first-hand the perils of equating fitness with weight loss. Sam was at her thinnest while smoking and really unfit. Tracy came to the FB50 Challenge with a mistrust of dieting and a history of yo-yo weight loss and gain. Weight and BMI just weren't going to cut it in determining what we meant by "fit." And most people would benefit from recognizing a wider range of available measures to inject more diversity into their fitness goals.

What Are You Made Of? Body Composition

Okay, so we decided that, for us, weight couldn't be a good measure of fitness. Those gold medal Olympic athletes whose BMIS put them in the overweight and obese categories must be all muscle. But even if we rejected BMI and weight as our FB50 goals, we could still look at our lean mass to fat ratio, or body fat percentage, a.k.a. *body composition*. Was an improved ratio, lean to fat, a goal worth pursuing?

During the course of our two-year challenge, we both tried to change our body composition. We sought out sports nutritionists and paid for online nutrition coaching. We both wanted to ramp up our food quality along with our increased activity and to make choices that better supported our very active lifestyles. But it's hard to keep separate a concern for visible abs as an aesthetic goal with improved lean to fat ratios for sports performance reasons. In the end, sad to say, it may be as elusive a target as weight loss.

How much do athletes care about body composition? It's everything in some sports—fitness competitions, for example—and almost meaningless in others. Some sports have specific weight and body composition goals needed for competition but the athletes don't expect to maintain those weights or lean mass to fat ratios throughout their training. Lightweight rowers and fighters talk about "making weight" for their events, but they don't stay there. Cyclists might have a racing season body fat percentage, but outside of serious racing season, it drifts up.

For the average, not naturally thin person, a low body fat percentage is not all that attainable—and maybe even not all that healthy. Yes, it's connected to concerns about physical fitness, and yes, it matters for some kinds of sports competition. But we each rejected it as a measure for our FB50 Challenge. One big motivator for us was that, over time, we came to see that there were loads of other ways to measure fitness, and they were frankly more fun.

Let's Get (un)Physical: Attitude and Mental Health

Why confine fitness to *physical* fitness? Lots of people take a more holistic approach. Attitude can have as much an impact on our quality of life as physical health. This isn't only about having a good attitude, but about developing the capacity for resilience, and even sometimes for suffering (cyclists like to talk about their ability to suffer), as markers of increased fitness or athletic capacity. And there's also evidence that regular activity can help fend off things like depression.

One of the things both of us consider non-negotiable is that, on balance, we need to enjoy the activities we pursue. Put up your hand if you've ever slogged through workouts as means to an end such as weight loss or fat loss. It's not that we never push beyond our comfort zone—for marathon training, Tracy has been known to drag herself out the door to run for two and half hours on an icy pathway in subzero temperatures. One memorable winter training session found her battling through the final five kilometres and suffering knee pain every time her right foot touched the ground. And she couldn't keep her hands warm even though she tucked them into her sleeves and wore gloves. That's all part of training. When we're doing things we love, we let the push that yields the war stories drive us forward some days.

One woman wrote to the blog to tell us that we could say what we like, she hates it all. She lamented that she did not and could feel passionate about a single activity in the whole wide world. What all had she tried? We don't know. But if she had truly given it an honest go and tried everything from ball hockey to tennis, from cross-country skiing to speed walking, then she's a rare and unfortunate exception. Most people can find some sort of physical activity that they either take to right off the top or that, over time and with some perseverance, makes their life more joyful and rewarding.

Another way attitude is relevant is in how we think about ourselves. Women who go through their lives hating their bodies, punishing themselves with fad diets, and berating themselves with harsh inner dialogue make us sad. It sounds so simple and cliché, but if you wouldn't talk to a friend that way, why would you talk to yourself that way? No good reason. Let's stop. It takes some work to revise the inner dialogue, but it pays off with a big return.

Meditation, especially mindfulness practices like body scanning and following the breath, develops a healthy attitude. Of course the Buddhist practice of mindfulness is hardly new. In fitness it has all sorts of applications, from mindful eating to mindful running. When we observe and detach from our emotions, choices, and physical condition rather than get caught up in them, we can translate challenges into opportunities to learn about ourselves. That knowledge can then be put to good use.

The only thing about using attitude as part of your fitness goals is that you can't jump on the scale or pull out a tape to measure it. It's just not trackable in the same way as some of the other indicators.

But we can check in with ourselves about attitude. Sometimes we need to remind ourselves or have others remind us about the fun factor. Not fun, ever? Then why do it at all? Tracy has really had to do a lot of soul-searching about cycling, which far surpassed running as her least favourite part of triathlon. She didn't mind it on race day, but the hours of training just filled her with dread. In the end, she made a commitment to focus on the bike, convinced that if she could see some performance improvement, she would like it more. But before she could do that, she had to get honest.

The same can be said about mindfulness and about attitude in general. If you commit to sit down and eat mindfully, then pay attention to what you're doing. If you become aware that you're planning your day instead of mindfully sipping your green smoothie, rolling the liquid around in your mouth, taking note of the coolness and how it feels on your teeth and tongue, then you just need to refocus your attention. Similar to gaining skills in sports, we can get better at mindfulness with practice even if we're not measuring and tracking stats.

Having a good attitude about your activities is one thing. What about the actual mental health benefits of fitness? It's a well-documented fact that regular physical activity can boost mental health in all sorts of ways. From reducing stress to releasing those feel-good endorphins, exercise can make us feel mentally better. People say exercise helps them feel more relaxed and less anxious. It's been credited with increasing brain power, sharpening memory, preventing cognitive decline, and even helping to control addiction.[2]

Do What You Love and Take It from There

If you decide (as we did) that fitness is more about what your body can do than about what it looks like, your list of options expands. You can choose from among a wide range of activities and sports with different goals. This happy diversity of possibilities prompts some people to say that there is no such thing as "fit," there's just "fit for a particular activity." After all, in cycling, hill climbers aren't sprinters. A really fit hill climber will look different from and perform differently than a sprinter. The sprinters in the Tour de France struggle to make it up the mountains. They're built for explosive speed, not climbing. When you move between sports, it gets harder still. You can't train for a marathon and build very much muscle. Bodybuilders limit their cardio so as not to detract from their lean mass.

We embarked on the FB50 Challenge with a shared view of fitness as something that includes strength, cardiovascular endurance, flexibility, balance, and coordination. We also included the more ephemeral measure of a sense of well-being. We weren't about to endorse any approach that pushed us to pursue things we hated and that didn't make positive contributions to our quality of life. We continued to think of fitness as varied in these ways as a base level from day one. Our FB50 Challenge pushed us each into different specialties and, on multiple measures, into becoming the fittest we'd ever been in our lives.

Take it away . . .

There are lots of different ways to measure your progress on the road to better fitness. If you take anything away from this chapter, let it be that the best approach will not be one-dimensional but will incorporate diverse indicators.

Try this . . .

If you have tended to focus on one area of improvement to measure your fitness, try adding another that you haven't consciously focused on before. For example, some people strength train, and are able to track increases by the simple fact that they can lift heavier weights than they could before, but they don't do anything for cardio health. If you're one of those people, think about rounding out your goals with some cardio training. Similarly, a runner might benefit from adding yoga. A yogi might benefit from a structured walking routine.

SIX

Love Your Body Now

Moving beyond Body Hatred, Food Deprivation, and Yo-Yo Dieting

NORTH AMERICAN women hate their bodies—not all of us, but anywhere from 50% to 91% of us, depending which study you read. *Quelle surprise.* The media and film industry present us with representations of an increasingly unattainable feminine body ideal. When we measure ourselves against the ideal of size zero celebrities, tall and thin runway models, or, even worse, digitally altered images in which even the original women don't look like that, we fall short. Comparison with others can make us feel bad about ourselves. It's easy to say that we should just reject the pressure to look a certain way. But the social expectation to conform doesn't come just from the media. Friends and family, healthcare professionals, and trainers and fitness instructors try to "help us" get or stay thin, with questions such as "Are you sure you should be eating that?" or "How much do you weigh this week?" We internalize these messages and learn to monitor and hate our bodies.

Body hatred and shame divert our attention from the things that really make us happy and rob us of a genuine connection to real sources of joy in our lives. If you're like many women, us included, you've spent at least some part of your life chasing an impossible ideal of thinness. Sometimes you might even have got there ... at least for a while.

Where Are the Women? Body Image, Gender, and Sport

On our blog we're amazed at how popular posts about body image are. Sometimes we even get bored or frustrated with the topic. Can't we just set body image aside and focus on sports performance and fitness more generally? And then another story about how body image affects fitness participation crosses our newsfeeds and we remember. Here's just one example. According to a BBC report on a campaign to get women more active, women are less likely than men to become active because of body image and competency fears. Research by Sport England shows "a significant gender gap, with two million fewer women than men in the 14–40 age range regularly participating in sport."[1]

Do those numbers shock you? They shock us. Here's another one: The mental health charity Mind found 9 in 10 women over 30 are afraid to participate in outdoor exercise. As a result, Mind began a campaign to encourage women to overcome the barriers such as self esteem that can harm their spiritual and mental well-being.[2] Other studies show that more than half of women won't take part in certain sports, such as cycling and rowing, because they fear the way their body looks in the form-fitting clothing associated with those sports. Lots of women say they exercise at night—like go for a run after dark—so no one will see them. In some neighbourhoods, that choice trades off physical security against body insecurity.

Another report from England talked about women actually running on treadmills in backyard sheds for fear of being seen and judged. The report was produced after Public Health England revealed once again the gender gap between women and men in hitting the recommended levels of physical activity: 31% of women engage in sport weekly versus 40.1% of men. The report, from the UK Commons' Health Select Committee, labels "fear of judgement" as a key factor for women's sub-par fitness levels.

As Sport England's Kay Thomson says, "Three quarters of women want to become more active but something is stopping them—fear of judgement. Judgement about appearance when exercising, ability to be active, confidence to turn up to a session, or feeling guilty about going to be physically active or doing something when you should have been spending more time with your family."[3]

Body image anxiety keeps women away from activity. Here's the common chorus: *I can't go to the gym. I'm too fat!* Women, small and large, miss out on the health benefits and the joy that comes from physical activity, either because they mistakenly think they're thin and don't need to exercise, or they think they are too fat to be seen out in public.

The gap between men and women in terms of physical activity starts early. According to StatsCan's 2015 Participaction Report, only 7% of Canadian children get the recommended amount of physical activity but that number hides a gender difference: 9% percent of boys but only 4% of girls meet the guidelines. That's sad. Physically active girls are much more resilient in terms of body image. Physical activity and sports participation protect young women from eating disorders.

The effect of body image on exercise starts young and doesn't stop when we get older. We saw earlier that only a small minority of women aged 50 or older feel okay about their bodies—just 12.2%. And rather than spurring people on to exercise, body dissatisfaction can keep them away from it because they worry they're "too fat" to be seen exercising in public.

The Quest for Body Beautiful

Body image is connected to fitness in other ways as well. Lots of women pursue physical activity with the sole motive of changing their bodies. We all know someone (maybe you *are* that someone) who approaches it like this: *I'll solve my body image issues by improving my body!* They start working out but don't lose weight, and then quit because they think getting thin is the sole point of exercise.

The quest for the body beautiful puts a huge amount of pressure on women. One area where we can see how the stakes have changed is in attitudes about the post-baby body. Sam has noticed that today there is incredible pressure to look good after childbirth, a pressure that she didn't experience—and her children, teenagers now, weren't born that long ago. No one ever expected her to be back in shape weeks or months after each of them was born. In her day, the idea of getting in shape between pregnancies seemed kind of like making a bed when you have an afternoon nap planned. Now new mothers are told that they are "letting themselves go" if they aren't back to their pre-pregnancy weight within six weeks.

What's changed? Celebrity culture, for one thing. From baby bump to the first torso pics after birth, we follow the lives of celebrity mothers. Some of us watch in awe at the transformations they undergo. And then there are post-baby cosmetic surgery packages that offer "mommy makeovers." And they're not just bellies and tummy tucks—now there's vaginal rejuvenation and labiaplasty as well. And don't forget the mommy-and-baby boot camps mobbing our parks on spring and summer mornings. Babies, outside exercise, company, and fresh air... Sounds like a winning recipe. But it's the "boot camp" part that is the problem. We've talked to friends who've taken part, and they felt whipped— almost shamed—into shape, in true "boot camp" style. They didn't like it at all. They were miserable.

If new moms can't escape the pressure, what about the rest of us? As much as we'd like to separate out body image and self-esteem from athletic performance and joyful movement, our culture makes that nearly impossible.

The Difficult Truth: Diets Don't Work

All that body hatred skews our views about fitness. There are lots of ways to change our bodies, but the way that seems most in reach is by losing weight. How do we lose weight? We go on a diet, of course! You've done it. We've done it. The neighbour has done it.

But here's a sad truth that many of us find difficult to face: diets don't work. We don't mean that you can't lose weight on a diet. Of course you can—people do it all the time. Tracy freely discloses that she has lost the same 10 pounds over and over again. Maybe you have too. Losing is the easiest part. Maintenance, anyone will tell you, is where the rubber really meets the road.

You know the drill. On January 1st, when you commit to that new diet or rejoin your favourite weight loss program (because they love offering specials to "returning members"), you may hold out hope that this time will be different. We see this scenario repeat itself over and over, with heartbreaking desperation, in the lives of women we care about and women we don't even know.

But the research data—and the personal experience of millions—show that restricted diets designed for weight loss rarely (not *never*, but rarely) produce long-term results. Take Weight Watchers, a worldwide weight loss business that offers meetings, memberships, and a range of products not limited to food, earning the company over $5 billion annually. Despite its popularity, it's tough to feel encouraged when you look at the long-term results. Every dramatic "success story" that appears in the ww promotional material has a teeny-tiny "results not typical" disclaimer hidden somewhere in the small print.

Typical results wouldn't attract people in such large numbers. The program has a low rate of success in even reaching the goal weight, and a still lower success rate in maintaining that goal weight over time. Researcher Michael R. Lowe studied the most successful ww members, those who'd achieved lifetime status by reaching their goal weight and maintaining it for six weeks in a row.[4] Five years after reaching their goal weight, 50% had maintained only 5% of their weight loss. Let's make that concrete: if

10 people lost 20 pounds, then five years later, 5 of them would have maintained a weight loss of 1 pound. Among the same group, on average only about 16 % remained below their goal weight five years after reaching it. And remember, these are the members who successfully reached their goal and maintained it for at least six weeks ... and most of them did not have dramatic amounts of weight to lose in the first place. Not surprisingly, Weight Watchers isn't all that open about the probabilities of reaching goal weight and achieving lifetime membership status.

Besides proving dismal over time, low-calorie diets wreak physical havoc. They create a famine response in the body, harm the metabolism, make it difficult to find the energy to get active, induce feelings of deprivation and even depression, and aren't healthy or sustainable. Does any of this sound familiar to you? If so, then you've probably experienced physical damage from restrictive dieting.

One group of researchers followed contestants from Season 8 of the popular reality show *The Biggest Loser* for six years.[5] Many regained a lot of their lost weight. They maintained some weight loss over the years, though—a mean weight loss of about 12% of body weight, and 8 out of the 14 participants maintained at least 10% weight loss. They kept up high levels of physical activity and careful control of their food intake.

But the study revealed serious metabolic damage that the contestants never recovered from. We all expect that our metabolism will slow down when we diet. That part didn't surprise anyone. But for these people, it never went back to normal, even though they remained highly active. This is called *metabolic adaptation*. The body fights really, really hard to get back lost weight. All of the contestants in the study burn hundreds fewer calories per day than expected for men or women their size. The message seems to be that extreme dieting and weight loss permanently slow the metabolism.

Hold on a minute. What does that say to those of us, ever the optimists, who hope against hope that we can one day lose weight, keep it off, and not go hungry—without having to be ever vigilant? We can live with lifestyle change, but permanent metabolic damage suggests that the chances of any diet leaving us better off metabolically are (ahem) slim. Of course, lots of people have questioned how representative these findings actually are. Maybe the Biggest Losers did it wrong, people say. They lost too much, too quickly. They stopped exercising (but that's not true, and that's partly why the data is alarming).

The cruellest irony of all is that people who embark on diets—not just *The Biggest Loser* contestants—usually end up *heavier* in the long run. Among the research that confirms this outcome, Evelyn Tribole, a proponent of the "intuitive eating" approach and co-author of the book *Intuitive Eating,* reports that a UCLA team reviewed 31 different diet studies on the effectiveness of diets. Their conclusion? Dieting is not just a bad way to lose weight, it's also a consistent predictor of long-term weight gain.

The media sells dieting as a quick fix. Headlines promote fast and easy weight loss. One of our most popular posts on the blog has "Raspberry Ketone, Garcinia Cambogia, and Green Coffee Extract" in the title. Why so popular? Because people desperate for the latest weight loss miracle punch these terms into their search engines in the hopes that they'll land, once and for all, on a magic solution. "America's favorite doctor" has endorsed each of these so-called miracle products at some point on his daytime television show.

But like so many other fads, from the grapefruit diet to the banana diet, from Dr. Atkins's approach to the South Beach Diet, the results are temporary at best. For the millions of us who have spent decades yo-yo dieting our way up and down and back up again, this news should come as no surprise. And yet whenever we publish anything on the blog related to the ineffectiveness of diets, we face all sorts of resistance.

If you've spent years on the diet train, still holding out hope that the right remedy or the correct formula just hasn't come your way yet, you may not like what we're saying about the miserable success rate of dieting. Sounds grim, we know. We don't like it either, but we like lies even less. Does it have to be all bad? Of course not.

Frankly, if you want stay active, then you need to provide your body with adequate nutrition to maintain a high level of activity. When we're hungry all the time, we don't have enough in the tank for a vigorous walk in the park, an early-morning bicycle ride, or a game of soccer with friends, never mind the more serious training we need to do if we're aiming to participate in bike rallies, marathons, or triathlons.

So here's a possible upside. While dieting damages our metabolic health, eating enough can sometimes repair it. Some people have apparently boosted their metabolisms. Amber Rogers, the woman behind the blog Go Kaleo, surmises that most people should be more worried about failing to eat enough than about eating too much. Matt Stone outlines a plan to reverse metabolic damage in a series of books called *Diet Recovery*. Again, the focus of the recovery is eating more, not less.

No diet aimed at weight loss ever recommends that you eat more. "Move more, eat less" is a common mantra, but it's really hard to move more if you're eating as little as most diets would recommend.

We're frequently asked, "If diets don't work, then what?" We promote two alternative approaches to food on our path away from dieting and toward healthier eating: intuitive eating and sports nutrition. Both reject the typical "eat less, move more" diet mentality of severely restricted eating. Both work well in tandem with a third way, "habit-based nutrition," promoted by some online nutrition coaching programs, including Precision Nutrition, which we took turns committing to, each for one year, during our fitness challenge.

Back to Basics: Intuitive Eating

The notion of intuitive eating comes from nutritionists Evelyn Tribole and Elyse Resch, who first outlined its principles in the

book *Intuitive Eating: A Revolutionary Program That Works.*
According to Tribole and Resch, intuitive eaters "march to their
inner hunger signals, and eat whatever they choose without experiencing guilt or an ethical dilemma." This sets them apart from
dieters, who must avoid internal cues and respond only to the dic-
tates of whatever their latest "plan" says they're allowed to eat.
The authors believe that children are born as intuitive eaters but
that social messaging leads many people to develop an unhealthy
preoccupation with nutrition, weight loss, and food. The goal
of the book is to help people who, in their words, have "hit diet
bottom" to become intuitive eaters. It really hit home for Tracy,
offering a new way of thinking about her relationship with food
and her body. If you've ever experienced your body as a battle-
ground and dieting as the only artillery at your disposal, it might
resonate for you, too.

The approach provides a new way of thinking about our relationship to food and our bodies. These ten principles sit at its
core:[6]

1.   Reject the diet mentality.
2.   Honour your hunger.
3.   Make peace with food.
4.   Challenge the food police.
5.   Feel your fullness.
6.   Discover the satisfaction factor.
7.   Cope with your emotions without using food.
8.   Respect your body.
9.   Exercise: feel the difference.
10. Honour your health with gentle nutrition.

The first four principles help to change your diet mentality,
that one in which food is the enemy and needs to be controlled
and restricted to reach your ideal weight. Principles 5 and
6—"feel your fullness" and "discover the satisfaction factor"—
nudge us in the direction of a more intuitive relationship to the

food we eat. Principle 7 addresses the issue of emotional eating and offers alternative modes of self-care that are more success-ful. Principle 8 calls upon us to stop body-bashing. Instead, let's respect the body we have.

Principles 9 and 10 come last for a reason. The authors believe that both exercise and attention to nutrition can be used as covert ways of implementing "the diet mentality." Not only that, but many people with a history of dieting and food obsession have negative associations with exercise in particular. Tribole and Resch strongly suggest that people work with the first eight prin-ciples to become comfortable intuitive eaters and only then pay close attention to exercise and nutrition.

Lifelong dieters will feel a combination of fear and exhilara-tion as they switch from chronic dieting to intuitive eating. When Tracy jumped on board for a year during the FB50 Challenge, within a short time her fear gave way to a sense of freedom. Mind-fulness replaced the need to control. A focus on physical activity nudged aside her previous dependence on the scale.

Maybe intuitive eating is too scary for you. Or you might feel skeptical that you actually will reach for a healthy range of foods in just the right amounts at the appropriate times (that is, mostly in response to physical hunger). Or maybe you're with Sam, who thinks that if she only ever listened to what her body says, she likely wouldn't get enough macronutrients (protein, carbs, healthy fats) to support optimum performance in all of the ath-letic activities in her life. If any of those doubts about intuitive eating resonate with you, then sports nutrition may be the way to go.

Fill the Tank: Sports Nutrition

There is no one recommended way of approaching sports nutri-tion. The basic idea is simple: focus on athletics and performance rather than on controlling weight. It's also a radical idea for many women to think of food as fuel for working out, rather than working out to burn off excess calories. It is more about getting enough of the right stuff than it is about limiting what you eat. Typically endurance athletes fuel long efforts with carbohydrates, and those whose focus is strength training aim to consume more protein. In recent years high fat diets have come into vogue for all kinds of different sports. And all athletes consume high amounts of fruits and vegetables with the aim of assisting recovery and muscle repair.

Sports nutritionists pay less attention to the number on the scale. They care about how athletes feel and what their energy levels are like. They are more likely to care about lean muscle to fat ratio than overall weight. While a diet-based approach recommends drinking lots of water to stave off hunger, sports nutritionists talk about hydration for activity. They set out to offer an evidence-based approach to nutrition that looks at all aspects of what we eat and drink, including caffeine, supplements, vitamins, and minerals.

But no matter what specific approach they take, sports nutritionists all share one key idea: that the focus of any nutritional plan should be on maximizing sports performance. In order to do that, sports nutrition advocates focus on (1) eating the right amount and balance of macronutrients, that is, protein, carbohydrates, and healthy fats; (2) taking these in at the right times in relation to training (also known as *nutrient timing*); and, for the more serious among us, (3) finding your "racing weight," that is, the weight at which you are going to reach your performance potential.

You Can't Leave It, So Why Not Love It? (and Treat It Like You Do)

On the positive side of this conversation, putting changing your body to one side, what does it mean exactly to love your body on its own terms, as it is now? We love fitness and physical activity. Faster, fitter, stronger, more powerful—these are all goals we share. But Sam says she also loves the body she has now: "What does it mean to 'love' this body? I don't think it's perfect, aesthetically speaking. That's not what I mean at all. I could list its flaws—I spend enough time with other women to know how to do that—but I won't. I love my kids. I don't think they are perfect. I'm not talking about aesthetics and I'm not talking about perfection. I don't associate either of those values with love."

Can you associate loving your body with the activity of caring for your body? Love is an activity. When we love other people, we care for them. And it's in that sense that we ought to love our bodies. There's also a sense of awe and wonder at what our bodies can do (*Wow, I rode my bike 160 km!*) and a response to that awe and wonder with concrete action (*Great ride, now let's go for a massage!*).

The philosopher Ann Cahill describes the process of losing weight while at the same time refusing to loathe the body she used to have. She writes, "I don't look back at photos of myself from a year ago and shudder. That was a different body that I lived, with its own set of possibilities, practices, and abilities. And there are certainly cultural contexts where that body would be more useful and conducive to my survival than the one I'm living now. Come the apocalypse, those extra pounds would come in handy."[7]

There's so much self-hate and negative talk presented as motivation for fitness training, but we think that self-hate is a pretty rotten motivator. For Sam, thinking negatively about the way she looks makes her want to stay indoors, watch TV, and eat nachos for dinner with Fudgee-Os for dessert, preferably while wearing big, baggy, fuzzy PJs . . . not to hit the gym.

Here are three things that do inspire and motivate us to stay fit and get fitter:

1. We both love trying new physical activities, and having a very high level of general fitness means that we can try new sports and physical pursuits without worrying so much about the fitness barrier.

2. We've both come to like sports competition, and if we want to keep racing, we need to keep up. Often there aren't very many people in our age group, and our racing companions are sometimes 20 years younger than us. Fitness helps even the playing field.

3. We both want to stay active as we age. We've got our sights set beyond mid-life, into retirement days and beyond. That's much more motivational for both of us than the body-perfect women in those "fitspiration" images.

Take it away...

Diets don't work and that's okay because food is fuel and so much more. We can learn to love our bodies now by focusing on performance goals instead of aesthetic goals. And it's completely okay to be a beginner—we all have to start somewhere.

Try this...

If you gave up on the goal of weight loss, what would your life be like? Try to imagine living without the scale as a measure of success. What would it be like to talk to (and about) your body the way you'd talk to and about a good friend, not a despised enemy? Write about it. Chat with a friend. Imagine a different way forward.

SEVEN

Competitive? Who, Me?

HOW COMFORTABLE are you admitting that you like to win? The very idea of competition is more fraught for most women than for most men. Women are supposed to be agreeable and kind of, you know, reserved. But competitive women are in your face and out there, right up there with the guys. It's not ... feminine. Some people might go one step further and say that it's not *feminist* for women to be in competition with other women. We're supposed to join together in solidarity, remember? How can we do that if we're trying to beat one another?

But come on, now—we're talking about sports here. How effective are we going to be if we don't try to win? Playing games against people who aren't even trying is kind of frustrating, don't you think? And as women, we don't need to deprive ourselves of the thrill of victory. So admit it. Claim it. It's okay to want to compete and win. We're allowed to bask in the glow of victory. And we can do it with grace and compassion. Tennis icon Chris Evert says, "If you can react the same way to winning and to losing, that's a big accomplishment." What's the take-away here? Winning is great and all, but competing is not only about winning, and it's definitely not about crushing your opponent.

Who's the Competition? Where's the Fun?

Lots of us are finishers, not placers. But even if you're a finisher, like Tracy, you can have a sense of competition. We compete with ourselves. When your Couch to 5K or Ease into 10K app says you've covered more ground in less time at a faster average pace than you did last time, you probably feel like you've earned a victory lap. And you have.

People like to say a race is a competition against yourself, against your own personal bests. We were both fortunate because when we started our FB50 Challenge, neither of us had any trophies gathering dust on a shelf in the basement. The challenge would have been far more daunting if we were competing against super-accomplished past selves. It's not fair to compare the times of a 50-year-old who has been running her whole life to the times she achieved in her 20s.

Sam had a couple "past Sam" contenders as formidable opponents. Sam at 40 was thinner and, if we use running as a measure, fitter than Sam approaching 50. She's probably slower on the bike. (She's certainly not as strong or as muscular. Shhh.) Contender number two was past Sam after 10 months of training and racing on her bike in Canberra, Australia. She did lots of road races, time trials, and criteriums. (A criterium, or crit, is a fast-paced bike race around a closed course that rewards both speed and tactics. Cornering fast matters!) Those were very happy, and very fit, times doing her favourite thing. That's when she learned to love racing.

But what if you're just not very competitive? Tracy has always said she had no interest in competition at all, and that's why she'd never done any kind of race before our FB50 Challenge. She was all about yoga and walking before that. She associated biking with leisure. Running? Forget it.

But Tracy has since gotten into racing—not to win, or even to place, but to finish. She gets a rare thrill when she finishes in the top half. This is a bit of a mental challenge for someone who confesses she's a poor loser—she feels badly about herself when she loses in a competitive situation.

When she was a PhD student in a stressful doctoral program in philosophy, Tracy and her housemate used to take time out from their studies by playing backgammon. But instead of serving as a happy outlet from a difficult day, backgammon became a complicated context of emotional management. The winner couldn't just play her best, most strategic game and win. Instead, they started to try to gauge how the other was feeling. Was the trouncing making her upset? Would using the doubling cube just be an added cruelty? Sometimes the winner apologized for winning. Sometimes the pending loser had to bow out, also apologetically, because she'd had a rough enough day already, thank you very much. No one got to feel good.

And so kicked in Tracy's aversion to competition. It wasn't just about the backgammon. Competing drained her emotionally. If she won, she felt a mixture of joy and guilt. If she lost, she felt inferior and unworthy. Competition can churn up all manner of feelings. Maybe this sounds familiar to you? So we have to ask: Where's the fun in that?

During those last six months of the first year of our FB50 Challenge, Tracy found the new attitude about competition that we recommend for anyone who decides to compete. Being able to bench press more weight, clocking a faster 10K, or beating your last 200-metre swim time trial give performance goals that put us in direct competition with no one but ourselves. Tracy adopted that approach. And she was a really good sport about it.

Why Race If You're Not Going to Win?

If you've never tried racing, then you may still wonder, "Why race if you know you're not going to win?" You can compete against yourself and improve on your past performances without entering actual competitions. But lots of people take part in races they have no hope of winning. If you look at the hundreds of people out for a local 10K running race, you realize that very few of those people are out with winning as their goal.

It's true in all sports at almost all levels that only a few people have realistic chances of standing on the podium at the end. Think of how many riders there are in the Tour de France and how few are serious contenders for even winning one of the stages, let alone the overall race. And if you've watched the race coverage from the start of the Ironman triathlon, the number of swimmers in the water is astonishing. In events like these, for which people need to perform at a very high level to qualify, the majority of participants aren't contenders for the podium, even in the age group categories.

Here are some points that may change your mind if you're not convinced there is a place for races or other sorts of competitions in your active lifestyle:

1. *It's fun.* Racing is a ton of fun. Whether you most enjoy the training, being out there competing, or the music, snacks, and prizes after, at the level of recreational athletics, it's all about the fun. Races have an atmosphere that celebrates athleticism at many different levels.

2. *Races serve as training goals for people at all levels.* Some are just aiming to complete the distance while others are aiming to place well among people of the same age, or to place well overall. There is something about race day that brings out the best performer in people even if they aren't going to win or place. Both of us have done vo_2 max testing and have a sense of what training in different heart rate zones means. Sam has worn a heart rate monitor when criterium racing on her bike. The first time she did this she laughed out loud when she saw the data because she spent so much time in the red zone—you can guess what that means! That's something most of us just can't force ourselves to do for very long outside race situations. Even if you're "only interested in fitness," not in racing, it's good to remember that fitness requires pushing yourself. And chances are remote that you'll ever push yourself as hard in training as you do when racing.

So races provide opportunities for fitness breakthroughs. They also give some structure to your training as you build endurance, then speed, then both together, then taper off coming up to the race, and then race, recover, and rebuild. And don't mock the accomplishment of finishing a certain distance. Finishing *is* something to feel good about. Imagine or think back on your first 5K race. If you've never run that distance before, finishing a 5K is an achievement.

3. *Lots of events raise money for worthy charities.* You can pursue your fitness goals and support good causes at the same time. And there are lots of causes to choose from. The Run for the Cure is not the only charity race, even if it's one of the biggest. Look for races that support causes you believe in, on both national and local levels.

4. *You can be competitive with individuals even if your goal isn't to win.* You can still have "winning moments," when you pass someone you can't ultimately beat or come in for the finish alongside (or maybe even slightly ahead of) the person you had in your sights the whole time. Sam was once bike racing with a group of women and she had pegged certain people as her competition. One woman in particular used to beat her each time there was a road race (hills!), but then Sam would beat her each week on the crit course. They each enjoyed the friendly competition. And for Sam, knowing where her rival was in the field of bikes helped her know better where *she* ought to be. Sam finished first in only one bike race, but she often beat her usual competitor. The friendly competition spurred each of them on to ride faster. Tracy does the same thing when running. In a race, it's a great strategy to find someone who runs at about the same pace and then try to stay with them to the end, maybe even pass them when you come close to the finish line. That's how Ironman champion Mark Allen finally beat then dominant and seemingly unreachable champion Dave Scott at Kona in 1989.

5. *Team competition feels somehow different, and might appeal to those who are less competitive as individuals.* When playing a team sport, you can experience competition as a way of helping out teammates rather than setting back your opponents. Playing defence in soccer, Sam was competitive in that she kept players from the opposing team from taking shots on the net, but she experienced it much more as supporting the team than anything else. She loved the feeling of being part of a team and having a role to play.

As you can see, even if you have always thought of competing in an event as somehow not worth it if you're not going to win, competing has got its merits. Planning for a race has spurred many of us on not necessarily to win, but to give it our best.

Never Too Late, Never Too Slow: Racing Is for Everyone

Suppose we're right and there are good reasons for racing even if you don't have a realistic chance of winning. Are there any downsides to racing? Some friends say they might have enjoyed racing in their youth but now they're too old. They've grown up and put all the fun away. But that's like saying that sex is only for the young. We've got one kick at the can, one try at this life, and if something would have been fun when you were young, it's probably still fun now. (Like sex.) The Veterans Cycling Club in Canberra, Australia, requires a doctor's note in order to keep racing after age 75, and when Sam was a member on her sabbatical a few years back, she met several people in that category.

Other friends we've talked to about racing worry they might get hurt. And that's true, they might. But you also might get hurt sitting on your sofa for too long, or shovelling snow. Life is risky—no way around it. In the category of recreational racing, most people recognize that we aren't professional athletes and there's no sense risking injury unnecessarily. Some of the rules in masters and recreational racing reflect this. On the one dodgy corner on the crit racing course in Canberra—"collarbone corner" as it's known—race organizers decided not to allow passing through that bend. For that one short turn, the race is "neutralized" and riders are asked to hold their place. Before every race, the organizer announces to the participants, "Remember, we're not racing for sheep stations out there." In other words, we're out here for fun, not fortunes.

Does all this focus on fun and participation take the glamorous competitive edge off sporting competitions? You hear this complaint mostly about running. Participation in marathons is on the rise globally. A research project out of the Copenhagen Business School studied participation data and race results from 2,195,588 marathoners all over the world. It found that from 2009 to 2014, the participation rate increased by 13.25% worldwide—and by close to 155% in India and 254% in China. For quite some time, there has been the worry that since marathons have become more popular and "accessible," the average time to complete has gone up. That's because there are more people who are in it just to finish, not to win. And this really bothers some folks. It's hard not to hear a gendered edge to this complaint given that the biggest increases have been in the numbers of women running. Yet the Copenhagen study reports that in many nations, the average finishing times actually improved over the study period. (Not in Canada or the U.S., however, where the average finishing time is slightly longer than it used to be—if Tracy's experience of stopping to get her picture taken with Batman during the Around the Bay 30K is at all typical, that may explain some of the increase... We're having more fun!)

The debate over the popularity of these events that were once considered available only to accomplished athletes often takes the form of a disagreement about whether everyone who finishes a race deserves a medal or whether medals should be reserved for those who win. Some medal sticklers don't even like age group medals. They think age group medals and finishers' medals belong in the same camp (Camp No Way!). After all, winning in your age group isn't the same thing as winning overall, or *really* winning! In the minds of these self-appointed gatekeepers, it's only the fastest times overall that count.

But there's lots to love about age group competitions, whether it's the "kids of steel" in triathlon events or the 80-plus group of marathoners like Ed Whitlock. Some of the age groups are pretty competitive. Whitlock ran a marathon in 2:52.47 when he was 69, and he was still running at the age of 85, just a year before he died in March 2017. And of course there's Olga Kotelko, who started competing in track and field at the age of 70 and held over 23 world records in her over-90 age group. You may imagine a thin competitive field in the over-90 group, but there's still something more than just a little bit incredible about Kotelko's story, which you can read about in Bruce Grierson's *What Makes Olga Run?*

There are even some people who think regional races don't count, only international races. For any race, just about, there's someone who thinks it's not the real thing. Maybe only the Olympics and the Tour de France and the Ironman get to count for real. But that misses out on the value of athletic competition. Only a very small percentage of the people in the world are elite athletes. Recognizing non-elite athletic performance is a good thing because even those who don't win accomplish something worthy of recognition.

A (Slightly) Academic Reflection on Competition, Femininity, and Feminism

When we blog about fitness and feminism, we talk quite a bit about "normative femininity." At the risk of sounding too academic (common in our line of work!), that's just a fancy label for the feminine ideals that women are supposed to adhere to. Whether we conform or not, most of us have already internalized the list. You know the drill: we're supposed to be nurturing and caring, good listeners, selfless mothers and daughters, that sort of thing. Being competitive, wanting to beat others and win, just doesn't seem all that "feminine." It's a little bit too selfish and "me first" to be a part of the standard repertoire of ideal femininity.

Feminists challenge that set of ideals. If we all conformed to normative ideals of what it means to be feminine, we would be submissive, subordinate, selfless caregivers who always put ourselves last. And that's not a firm path to equality.

But some say competition also runs counter to feminist ideals. The very idea of competition, they say, is a feminist taboo. Feminists have had difficulty talking about competition because they consider it a key feature of the patriarchal social structure that feminists criticize. The default assumption that competition is not just unfeminine (though it is that too), but actually unfeminist, that it goes against the goal of equality. It's sometimes bad, and sometimes downright ugly.

Competition isn't just suspect for being masculinist and patriarchal (and capitalist). It's divisive and hierarchical. That's where it runs up against equality. You can't have winners without losers. And aren't winners superior to losers? The gold medalist stands at the top of the podium. What about feminist solidarity? What about equality? How does a good feminist reconcile competition with that?

This unease with the idea of competition means that many women who consider themselves feminists are loathe to admit to their competitive tendencies. Here's how they see the world (maybe you can relate): We compete with ourselves. We support our sisters. We hold hands as we cross the finish line.

And yet, feminist or not, feminine or not, don't we all like to win?

Tracy likes to tell the story of playing Scrabble with a friend who didn't care about winning. She just played any old word, not striving to lay down all the tiles, land on triple word scores, or get the most out of blanks and Qs and Zs. That's not how Tracy plays Scrabble. Where she comes from, you play to win. You challenge words. You play by the rules. You do not—let's be really clear about this— do not, under any circumstances, leave an open triple.

Sam played for a masters women's soccer league that kept score during games but didn't record the results anywhere. Some people didn't even want to tally up the points at all. But even if you're playing for fun, surely trying to score goals and beat the other team is part of what makes team sports fun, isn't it? It's part of what makes them sports.

Whether in Scrabble or in soccer, even if you win, it's hard to feel like a winner unless both sides are competing. Playing with someone who doesn't care is just one step short of playing with someone who lets you win. It's tough to get worked up about empty victories handed over on a silver platter. That's not how competition works.

There's an ugly side to competition, of course: envy, jealousy, resentment. We want to feel happy for our friends who succeed, but instead we sometimes envy their success, wishing it were ours. And then we feel guilty for feeling that way.

If you've lived on both sides of the envy, you know that neither feels good. When you care about your friends and know that your successes in some way hurt them, then it's easy to feel hurt in turn (*Why aren't they happy for me?*). And since you do care, you then have to downplay your victories and successes (like not keeping track of the standings in Sam's soccer league, because God forbid that one team should outplay the rest consistently *and we keep a record of that!*).

But let's think about this for a minute. Aren't sports perhaps the one domain where women can compete against one another in a healthy, socially acceptable way? What a relief to have an area in life where we don't have to be nurturing and cooperative and all concerned about whether our success is making someone else feel bad!

In sports, if nowhere else, we can go for the win because that's what it means to play. We can feel empowered at our own accomplishments while at the same time applauding the success of those who train harder or have done better in the genetic lottery than we have. We can set ourselves personal goals and, as Sam likes to do, look at ourselves as our fiercest competition. We can admire champions.

If you're a woman who has experienced some discomfort with the idea of competition—perhaps for reasons you're clear about, perhaps for reasons you're not so clear about—you may find that sports and athletics let us find the good in competition. Mariah Burton Nelson gives a feminist take on victory in sports in her engaging and accessible book *Embracing Victory: Life Lessons in Competition and Compassion, New Choices for Women*. It's really about winning with grace and compassion, about developing your own measures of success (and not necessarily shying away from winning as a goal), about attending to the process, about being willing to lose.

Let's give ourselves permission to compete. Lift the taboo and lighten up.

We don't have to hold hands across the finish line. But we can go for the group hug when we all get there.

What about Competing for Weight Loss?

If competition is a healthy thing that can help us feel good about ourselves, does that extend to weight loss competitions? Competitive weight loss came under the spotlight (and the microscope) with the popular television series *The Biggest Loser*. Weight loss competitions based on this reality TV show have since sprung up in gyms and offices all over the Western world. Every year when winter folds into spring, you probably see big signs in front of studio windows or in gym lobbies with those typical dramatic before-and-after pairs of photos, advertising weight loss competitions. Maybe you've even joined in on one, thinking it would be a good way to motivate a committed weight loss effort.

But these don't fall into the category of healthy competition.

Apart from the fat-shaming and abuse that people have come to expect from the show (maybe they're even the reason so many tune into the show), the whole idea of a weight loss competition buys into a set of cultural attitudes that we all need to challenge. Maybe it's news to some, but guess what: different people lose weight at different rates. Let's say you enter a weight loss competition that runs over a 12-week period. You can be sure that the amount of weight various people lose won't necessarily track effort even if we were to measure the loss in terms of percentage of starting weight rather than absolute numbers on the scale. And did the people whose before-and-after photos they use to recruit others make those changes in just 12 weeks? Probably not. Before-and-after photos can be misleading in all sorts of ways.

It's just sad to pit people against one another like this over weight loss. Can you relate to the horror of weigh-ins with personal trainers or weight loss program counsellors? It can feel demoralizing even when we're not competing against anyone. Adding the element of competition, including material rewards and prize money, raises the stakes. If weight loss is the focus, you can be sure that diet is going to play at least as important a role as the workouts. They'll be recommending restrictive eating plans. Let's call them "diets." And the jury's back—yes, back—with their verdict on that whole issue: diets don't work.

Plus the focus on weight loss can, if not done responsibly, have a damaging effect on your metabolism. The study of the Season 8 participants, which we mentioned in the previous chapter in our discussion of dieting, painfully bears this out. The research shows that most of them are burning hundreds of calories less per day than would be expected for a man or woman of their size. Keep in mind that this is years later, not just immediately after the weight loss. Their metabolisms simply did not recover.

Weight loss is not the only measure that we should be attending to, folks. For one thing, it's possible to improve fitness without losing weight, even with gaining weight. If your body composition changes, then you may experience no weight loss at all yet be stronger and even leaner. And you don't even have to change your body composition to benefit from activity.

The idea of entering a competition to see how much weight you can lose might seem motivating and exciting at first, but the fact is it ends up making most of us feel like crap.

Yes, yes, we know: it's a reality of our time that people want to lose weight, will pay big bucks to do it. But still and all, even though we believe in competition, weight loss competitions are just a bad idea.

Take it away...

As feminists, we don't have to deprive ourselves of opportunities to compete. Competition has all sorts of rewards besides winning. Race day has its own kind of adrenaline rush, and team sports have lots to offer. Setting personal goals and trying to beat your past self can motivate improved performance. And if you can feel the same way about winning as about losing, you've got the right kind of attitude to get the most out of competing.

Try this...

Pick a competitive event, gather up some friends, sign up, train together, and commit to a fun day out whether you win, lose, place, compete, or complete.

EIGHT

The FB50 Challenge

Six Months to One Year— Tracy's and Sam's Stories

March to August 2013

Tracy's Story: Triathlon, a Love Story

The story of the next six months is about falling in love with triathlon as I prepped for the Kincardine Women's Triathlon. I approached the event as a one-off, the way you might think of a thing to check off of the bucket list. The KWT is a small event— fewer than 300 women—friendly to newbies, with a very short course. If you have it in your life plans to do a triathlon, Kincardine may be the most fun, least demanding way of meeting that goal. For most of the course you are right on the shore of Lake Huron, except, of course, for the swim, when you're actually in it. I knew Kincardine, Ontario, with its picturesque harbour and charming lighthouse, as a stop along the way from Bayfield, where we kept our sailboat, up to the North Channel, our favourite summer sailing destination, in Lake Huron north of Manitoulin Island.

I took some comfort in knowing that the KWT was a women-only event with a strict limit on the number of participants. Have you ever seen the television footage of hundreds of swimmers crawling over one another at the start of a triathlon? I could just imagine being pulled under, kicked in the head, or crowded out of contention.

But that was all months away, right?

March to April 2013: Making a Splash

With my Y membership in hand, I savoured my time in the pool. I'd loved swimming since childhood. My mother forced us into lessons because taking advantage of the freedom to take swimming lessons affirmed our new life as immigrants in Canada. My homeland of South Africa denied lessons to anyone non-white. As a family in Cape Town classified as "Coloured" under the South African race segregation system of apartheid, that ruled us out. Maybe that's why I always experience a surging sense of freedom when I dive into a lake, a pool, or the ocean.

Swimming put some rhythm and structure into my "training." It's not as if I trained hard, like an athlete, in the months leading up to Kincardine. Instead of serious training, the next six months would be a period of challenge and discovery.

A major change in my approach during that time was that weight loss no longer served as my primary motivation. Remember, I'd stopped weighing myself on January 1, the same day I signed up for the triathlon. With that off my mind, I had more mental space for other things.

In March and April, those other things were running, swimming, yoga, and weight training. You'll notice that cycling doesn't make this list. I stayed in denial about the biking part of triathlon almost until the day of!

When you're a new triathlete—when you hesitate even to call yourself a triathlete—everyone tells you not to worry, you can ride any kind of bike. No need for a dedicated triathlon bike (I had to wonder, "What does a triathlon bike even look like?"). Sam assured me that in this all-ages, -shapes and -sizes event, I'd see people on commuter bikes, mountain bikes, and bikes with baskets and flowers on them, as well as racing-style road bikes and triathlon bikes. My hybrid would do the trick well enough to let me see whether there would be more triathlon in my future. And since, months ahead of the event, I didn't foresee triathlon in my future—this was just a lark for the blog, remember?—it didn't make sense to invest in anything fancier.

So: running, swimming, yoga, and weight training. For each, I had to decide how frequent and when. At this stage in the challenge, with my ultimate goals still ill formed, yoga continued to take priority. Everything else had to work around it. I had my Tuesday-morning Iyengar yoga class each week, and an unlimited pass for hot yoga at another studio, both within walking distance of where I lived. The unlimited pass worked for me then in a way it would not in the months to come once I got more serious about multisport training. Unlimited passes, like all-you-can-eat buffets, create built-in incentive to do more. At first, I got my money's worth with at least four hot yoga classes a week, and some weeks I went to five or six. Being on sabbatical for the year—a year off from undergraduate teaching responsibilities to focus on research and writing, one of the major perks of academic life—helped too. Sabbatical years are the only times I've ever felt I really have enough time for writing, working out, and catching up with friends without having to sacrifice sleep.

I ran regularly but didn't "train." I had nothing against training, but I really didn't know how. My only goal was to keep increasing my distance through that first winter of running. That winter was relatively mild, but still, I had never experienced winter running. I worried over the cold. I feared slipping on ice. When I went into a local running shop to buy some winter gear, I felt completely at sea. I bought some thicker tights and a couple of long-sleeved tops but didn't even own a running jacket. I adopted a simple strategy: walk-run intervals, and if it snowed, I stayed home (because no jacket!).

I think back on those months as leisurely and relaxing. Panic over the upcoming triathlon hadn't yet set in.

May and June 2013: Picking Up the Pace

That all changed in May. You know what it's like: you commit to something months away, and it feels so harmless. But when the snow melted and the magnolias began to bloom, the July triathlon just didn't seem that far away anymore.

And the thing is, everyone was starting to *know* we were doing Kincardine. Most people don't know the difference between an Ironman and anything else. They hear "triathlon" and they think Kona, in Hawaii—the birthplace of the Ironman and admittedly the beginning of the trend toward the swim-bike-run endurance event.

Kona is a 2.4 mile ocean swim followed by 112 miles on the bike and then a marathon (26.1 miles). Kincardine is no Kona. We're talking a 400-metre swim, 12 kilometres on the bike and a 3-kilometre run. When I look on it now, I see it's something most people in reasonably good condition can finish with no training at all.

But I didn't know that then. And not many of the people around me did, either. Whenever I said I was doing a triathlon in July, people almost always said, "Wow!" I tried to downplay the prospective "achievement" (not yet an achievement of any kind) by reminding them that it would be "just a small triathlon." But no matter—impressed they remained.

After a winter without bike training (and no idea what bike training would even look like), I continued into the spring with very little time on my bike. Being on sabbatical, I had no need to go to campus, which is my usual regular ride, about 4K each way. It still hadn't really sunk in that training might be a good idea. It's astonishing to me now how ignorant I was about preparing for a race. My workouts up to this stage of my life had never been designed to *prepare* me for anything. They'd been totally geared toward weight loss and "toning."

There's a lot to think about when you start to plan for a triathlon. I had no conception of intervals on the bike or which gears to use or how to go faster. My bike had flat pedals, not clipless, so I couldn't even get the maximum power from my pedalling. None of this even entered my mind until later in June, when Sam encouraged me to get out for a ride on the bike path. I rode 11K with her that day, the farthest I'd gone on my bicycle, possibly ever, certainly in decades. I remember feeling nervous and tired. Cycling is a different kind of endurance. But at least I did it, and I knew I could do it on race day.

For the first time that spring, I joined a learn-to-run clinic through a local shop. I knew so many people who trained in groups, from running to biking to swimming, but except for my weight training in the mornings with Renald and the yoga classes I attended, to that point I'd undertaken all of my activities in solitude. Nothing against solitude, but it turns the activity into more of a meditation than a challenge. I like to meditate. There's something to be said for repetitive activities that bring on a meditative state. Some of my best writing ideas come when I'm swimming or running. I even used those activities (or walking) as strategies when I felt stuck in my writing. But I wasn't necessarily challenging myself physically, and I still felt like a really inexperienced new runner.

I joined the learn-to-run clinic hoping to up my performance game. We met every Wednesday at the back of the running shop, squeezing ourselves in among the sale racks stuffed with last season's gear, for a little talk about gear or injury or how to choose the right shoes for your foot and your gait. And then we broke out into groups and ran. My clinic had three levels—total newbies, who did a walk-run combination; level twos, who ran continuously, adding a few minutes each week until eventually making it to 28 minutes of continuous running; and the level threes, who seemed to me not even to be "learning" anymore, because they started with 20 minutes without a break on the first day. At the time that seemed impossible to me—I'd only done it once, way back in September.

I had a great moment on the very first day of the clinic, before we even set out for our first very short run. The clinic leader went around the room and asked us what we were doing there, and what we hoped to gain from the next few weeks. My answer: I wanted to get more comfortable running without needing walk breaks, I wanted to get faster, and I wanted a sense of community, maybe even to meet people I might continue to run with when the clinic ended. What's missing from that list? Weight loss! Wanting or expecting to lose weight didn't come up even once during my little schpiel.

We all have our epiphany moments. I'd set aside the scale and turned to intuitive eating, trying to let my appetite and my body be my guide. On that first day of the clinic, I stood in the back of the running shop amid the shelves of neon shoes and the racks of shorts and the displays of socks with a group of eager new runners. When performance and community were the first two reasons I had for wanting to join a running group, it hit me as my first huge breakthrough of the Fittest by 50 Challenge.

My attitude was, indeed, changing.

July and August 2013: Before You Know It, It's Race Day!

If you've ever signed up for anything that a little voice in the back of your head (or a big voice with a megaphone in front of your face) told you you couldn't do, you'll know the fear. That fear helped to fuel my focus on my performance. When June rolled into July, the "little" triathlon just two weeks away grew epic in my mind. I don't know about you, but I'm the type of person who likes to be informed. I also procrastinate. That combo meant I consulted far and wide about how best to prep, but that I waited until the last two weeks before the event to do so. Because I have great friends who are generous with their information, I received loads of it. Maybe too much.

Gone were the days when, in my ignorant bliss, I thought the only thing to be concerned about was training for three events. A little swimming here, some running there, with some cycling thrown in. Not so bad.

But no. Once the reality of triathlon sets in, you learn in swift order that training for the three events is *not* all there is to it. Two enormously important things to which I'd remained completely oblivious until that July were clothing selection and, the scariest thing of all, the transitions, a.k.a. T1 and T2.

I've seen photos of intense-looking people running from the water to the transition area, barefoot with their wetsuits pulled down around their waists. I read somewhere that it's a good idea to visualize the transition. See yourself running from the water to your station, removing your wetsuit (another thing I hadn't thought about), drying off, pulling on your shorts, putting on your shoes, sunglasses, and helmet, getting the bike ready, hopping on, and going.

But if you've never even seen a transition area, it's really hard to picture all that. To put this in context, a couple of years later, when I was a seasoned triathlete and we coaxed a friend into trying Kincardine for the first time (that's a thing with us, luring friends into our activities so we can spend more time with them), she thought the transition area would be in a barn. How in the heck is an inexperienced newbie supposed to know? And unlike the Ironman, there would be no "wetsuit peelers" at the swim-to-bike transition to help us peel the suits off. Was peeling off the suit even the most challenging part of T1?

I may be self-taught, but I like to learn. If you're considering triathlon, here's what I learned from my voluminous sources. The key to a good transition is to have your own little area set up properly, for maximum efficiency. An experienced triathlete can do the swim-to-bike transition in less than a minute, bike to run in less than 30 seconds. But in less competitive rosters, the average times are much longer—2 minutes for the swim-to-bike, 45 seconds for the bike-to-run.

Each competitor has a small space where they rack their bike and can set up their stuff. Hang the helmet on the handlebars with the open side up, sunglasses inside with arms open, ready to be put on. If you have a water bottle for the bike, put it in its holder. If it fits, place a towel, folded in half, on the ground beside the bike. So far I've never been to an event where there was no space. Shoes on the end of the towel, laces open or elastic quick-tie laces in, socks tucked loosely into shoes. T-shirt should be on the towel with the race number pinned onto the front of it (or have a race belt—not yet part of my world at that first triathlon, but a definite one now—on the towel, number attached). You'll want another towel for a quick dry-off after the swim.

My head spun. Why? This setup requires a number of apparel decisions. Do I go with the quick-tie laces? I initially thought that since I'd be zooming along on my city bike with its flat pedals and wouldn't have to change from bike shoes to running shoes in T2, I might just stick with my regular laces. Maybe that might even give me a competitive edge over the people who have to take the time to change their shoes. Apparently, the answer is no. Someone alerted me that lace tying can be an issue when you've come out of the cold lake. Your fingers just aren't as dexterous as usual, and tying shoelaces can be a frustrating challenge. So yes: elastic laces. Or, as I do today, regular laces already tied, with a shoehorn at hand so I can slide my feet into my shoes and be done with it. (I'm the only one I've ever seen doing this, so I'm not saying it's a widely documented race-day strategy, but it works for me).

What to wear under my wetsuit and what to change into? Having no idea what my future held on the triathlon front, I could not justify investing in any special clothing like a triathlon suit (other than the laces). The weekend before (!!) I did a wetsuit test run with my running bra and running undies under the suit. It felt comfortable and it was easy to swim. But do people really strip down to underwear and then pull on shorts in T1? I can answer that now: no.

Even the decision to wear a wetsuit is crucial. I'd never considered a wetsuit until I read on the race page that you could rent one. Sam told me that her biggest mistake in a previous triathlon was not trying out the wetsuit ahead of time. I considered forgoing the wetsuit, but the race page for our triathlon kept noting the water temperature in Kincardine as "COLD!!" with no actual temperature. It was like that all winter, but by July 2, just two weeks before the event, it still said that. I only had a scuba wetsuit.

How different could it be? I had worried about mobility and how it might affect my stroke. On the test run the week before, I had no problem with mobility in the suit, but I could surely attest that Lake Huron is c-c-c-c-cold.

A week prior to the event, here's where things stood gearwise: Wetsuit—CHECK. Quick-tie laces—CHECK. Running underwear—CHECK. Old standby running shorts, shirt, socks, and shoes: CHECK, CHECK, CHECK, CHECK.

There is an order of actions at the transitions. My friend Chris shared a tip sheet that she got from her triathlon training group. It's two pages long, and to this day I hold that tip sheet responsible for my sense of panic as I realized how much there is to think about (but I still use it as a checklist). It's common sense that if the setup is good, the transition should go well. The tip sheet recommends leaving the goggles and swim cap on until you've finished stripping off the wetsuit at the bike. Step on the towel you've laid out on the ground to dry your feet. Pull on your socks and put the shoes on. (I would also have to remember to pull my shorts on first—but as you will see, it turned out on race day that the conditions saved me from myself. A tip for newbies: Always wear under your wetsuit what you plan to wear on the bike and the run.) Then the shirt, sunglasses, and helmet (CHIN STRAP DONE UP!!—*their emphasis*). You run your bike to the mount-dismount line, cross the line, mount, and ride. That's transition 1.

Transition 2 has its own complications. You have to get off the bike *at* the line—no riding through the line at your fastest speed like in a bike race. Take off the helmet, change your shoes if needed, grab your hat, and *run*.

That seemed straightforward enough. But then I read about "heavy leg syndrome." Running from a long bike ride is just not the same as running on its own, or starting from a warm-up walk. Here's what can happen, according to an article on Active.com about mastering the transition from bike to run: "Your free-flowing running gait, which was the hallmark of your style when you ran fresh, is reduced to nothing more than a pathetic shuffle as you struggle to maintain contact with those with whom three minutes earlier you were riding shoulder-to-shoulder."[1]

I followed the article's advice and started doing some "brick" training, another concept new to me until about two weeks before my Kincardine triathlon debut. In a brick workout you stack workouts back to back, following a bike ride with a run. And you know what? Your legs do feel funny. They want to keep going in circles, like on the bike. And they feel heavy, like someone poured lead into them.

Then there are all the little things. Spare goggles in case a strap snaps before the swim. Practising with the wetsuit. Learning to remove it as quickly as possible. I came across a list of dos and don'ts that included things like bring your own toilet paper; bring a bike pump; set yourself a pre-race visual cue, like a ribbon or a balloon or something on your bike, so you can find it quickly after the swim; take your time in the transition—which seemed counterintuitive, but it makes sense that rushing might lead to forgetting something crucial. And don't try anything new, bring too much, take up more than your allotted space (a major etiquette violation), or forget anything important. Only half of these even made sense to me, never having even set eyes on a transition area, let alone stepped foot in one.

All of that pre-triathlon information helped me and terrified me at the same time. In those days leading up to race day, I had to keep reminding myself: this is for fun. It was, after all, a "try-a tri." The whole point was to try something new and see if I liked it.

Still and all, the lead-up to the day of event was a nerve-racking time. I felt woefully underprepared for the cycling portion of the triathlon but knew I could finish the 12K ride. For all my running aspirations and fairly consistent training, I've never managed to sustain a good pace without needing walk breaks, not even for the 3K distance Kincardine asked of us. And though I was more than prepared to do a strong swim, even in mid-July and even with a wetsuit, the lake was mighty cold on the day of the race.

As it turns out, the lake temperature failed to meet official triathlon standards. That meant that on the morning of the event, just as I approached the bathing cap table to pick up the pink cap for the 45-and-overs, they announced that they'd made the difficult to decision to cancel the swim. The water was a chilly 10°C (50°F) and fell under the regulation minimum of 13°C with a wetsuit and 14°C without. Ugh!

Sam had already changed her registered event to the duathlon a couple of days before. My friend Tara was elated at the announcement because the swim was the part that was scaring her the most. But Sam's daughter, Mallory, and I were seriously bummed. Both of us, as strong swimmers, had been counting on the swim to get a head start. Neither of us felt enthusiastic about adding a second run.

In a duathlon you run-bike-run. Like the triathlon, it still involves two transitions. In the case of the Kincardine Women's Triathlon, the duathlon was a 3K run, a 12K bike ride, and a 3K run.

There was no way I was going to quit just because my strongest event had been cancelled. At least, unlike Mallory, who chose to do the whole thing in bare feet, I had shoes!

On that hot summer day in July, with a clear blue sky, the whole event took place along the water, along the eastern shore of Lake Huron. My husband and I had sailed up to start our summer vacation the day before and took a slip at the marina, right beside the event site.

We arrived pretty early, but lots of people were there already. The buzz and excitement fill the air at these things. I feel a real charge from the energy. A volunteer came around with a bike pump and offered to check my tires—a good thing, because they needed air.

The announcers at Kincardine did an exceptional job of providing non-stop information about transitions. I guess they figured the more they announce about not touching the bike until you had your helmet on and not getting on the bike until you got to the mount-dismount line, the less likely anyone would mess that part up. They were upbeat and encouraging.

In the portable toilet line I chatted with a few women about the cancelled swim. The swim clearly divided the competitors into two camps. Some were so relieved it surprised me that they hadn't signed up for the duathlon to begin with. The other half felt like I did—sad about missing out on their strongest event and a bit apprehensive about doing two runs.

We went in three waves: under 35, 35 to 44, and 45 and over. There were much more finely grained age categories, but at the starting line these three waves mattered. Mallory went in the first wave, then Tara three minutes later, then Sam and I.

You kind of get caught up in the thing, and before you know it, you're running. Then before I knew it again, I was taking a walk break. Then running again, then walking, and so on. By the time I got back to the transition point, there were hardly any bikes left—even fewer than I'd anticipated—but off I went on my commuter bike hoping to make up some lost time! Renald cheered me on from the sidelines.

Sam blasted past me on the bike around the 4K mark, but I did manage to pass a few women. Despite my concerns about the cycling portion, I enjoyed it the most, probably because I associate cycling with leisure (not the best race strategy, but I look back on that bike ride with a warm feeling). I really felt good on the bike and wished for more of a performance bike.

They say to start prepping for the run in the last part of the bike. My version of prep was to start obsessing about how I would even make it. A final brutal hill when there was about 1.5K left in the bike ride kept me in the moment, but at the bottom of that uphill I could clearly see the halfway point turnaround of the run. Women streamed past me on their way back, looking spry and game. For a brief moment I felt disappointed in my performance.

The final run challenged me. I ran alongside a few other women, walked a bit, and managed to keep running, albeit slowly, for the final kilometre by using positive self-talk. The volunteers and lots of wonderful onlookers cheered us on: *You've got this! You can do it! You're almost there! Keep moving!* I've come to know this secret: in the best events the community comes out to support the athletes, even the competitors at the back of the pack.

I felt amazing when I crossed the finish line. I wasn't the fastest person by any stretch, but it was the most demanding physical thing I'd ever done to that point in my life. Never before had I moved continuously like that for one hour and 22 minutes.

The age, size, and ability range of the women inspired me. Most amazing to me were the women in the 60+ categories who did this thing in an hour. An hour! I was still 48 at the time, and that gave me something to aim for and 12 years to do it. If I could shave off two minutes a year...

Kincardine turned me on to something new, and it had a hold on me from the minute we stepped into the park. There are things you don't know about triathlon or duathlon until you actually do it.

Like the body marking. They wrote our numbers (mine was 200) on our left arm and our ages and events on our right calf, in black marker. It made me feel really badass—like a real competitor. And it gave me perspective. At one point, a 62-year-old flew past me on the bike! A few other times, I passed women who were younger than me. I'm not a big comparer or a big competitor, but I liked knowing everyone's age.

And the timing chip, on a Velcro strap around the ankle. From the moment I strapped it on, I couldn't feel it. What I love about multisport events is that they don't just give you an overall time, you get a time for each portion, plus for your transitions.

And the energy in the air. Pre-race, the excitement mixed with apprehension creates a kind of intensity that gets the blood flowing and the heart pumping. Because of the time and care needed to get your transition area set up and to make sure everything is ready to go, it takes a different kind of focus than a single-discipline event.

The biggest bonus of the multisport model for me was how it let me train for endurance in a way that's not all about running. At that point in my life, I still thought running might not be my thing. That's evolved since the end of the FB50 Challenge, but in the early days, I had limited aspirations in that department because I associated running with injury. I still thought more along the lines of decent 5 and 10K times. Sticking to triathlon, when coupled with the two other events, those distances could give me an "endurance" experience of being out on the course for a couple of hours.

But one thing about the Kincardine Women's Triathlon that didn't go as planned: it wasn't a triathlon. I had to find an actual triathlon to get the full experience.

From Kincardine I sailed north on Lake Huron with Renald for our annual summer vacation on the water. The minute I got back in early August, I started to train for Lakeside's Give-It-a-Tri, a swim-bike-run within easy driving distance of home, held annually on the weekend after Labour Day.

I didn't have a whole lot of time to train, but I felt committed to giving the "tri" a try. Jolene, our athletic, game niece from Renald's side of the family, responded to my desperate plea on social media for company on race day. Jolene runs fast but had never trained for anything other than running.

My training during that month was haphazard and unfocused. I really didn't know what I was doing. I figured I should try to give equal time to swimming, biking, and running. But in the end, I kept up with running three times a week, swimming twice, and biking for leisure on the bike path.

My long-standing aversion to riding my bike on the road— verging on an all-out phobia that I would be hit from behind by a car—had a negative impact on my training. I could come up with all sorts of excuses not to go out. But the main excuse was: I didn't have the right kind of bike to train "properly." The easy answer to that is to buy a new bike. And at the end of August, that's exactly what I did. After some hemming and hawing about whether to buy a road bike or a tri-bike, I tried out a few road bikes at local bike shops and put in my order.

I may not have been well trained for the bike portion of Lakeside, but at least I was equipped.

TRACY'S TYPICAL TRAINING WEEK, MARCH–AUGUST 2013

MONDAY	7 A.M. WEIGHT TRAINING; 5 P.M. HOT YOGA
TUESDAY	6:30 A.M. IYENGAR YOGA; 11 A.M. SWIMMING AT THE Y
WEDNESDAY	7 A.M. WEIGHT TRAINING AND 5K RUN
THURSDAY	11 A.M. SWIMMING AT THE Y
FRIDAY	7 A.M. 5K RUN
SATURDAY	8:30 A.M. HOT YOGA
SUNDAY	8:30 A.M. HOT YOGA

What's wrong with this picture? Still no scheduled rest day!

Tracy's Events and Milestones, March–August 2013
- July 2013 The Kincardine Women's Triathlon, Kincardine, Ontario—changed to a duathlon due to water temperature

Sam's Story: From Jet Setter to Couch Jockey

While the first six months of the challenge went better than could be expected (a new belt in Aikido! winning an ergatta!), the second six months weren't such smooth sailing as I tried to deal with illness and work travel. It was also the period in which I added to the mix—because running, biking, rowing, Aikido, and CrossFit weren't enough—the burpee challenge. Rowing's new challenge was moving from the boathouse and the rowing machine to a nearby lake. I also started an online nutrition counselling program to help with fuelling all this movement.

Sickness and a Setback

Academic positions can involve a lot of work-related travel. We fly to conferences, workshops, and dissertation defences. We work with colleagues at distant universities too, so at a research-intensive university that adds up to a fair bit of flying around. When my children were little I limited myself to one out-of-province trip a month, but since they became teenagers and I stopped being department chair, I no longer had those excuses. The second term of this university year involved a lot of finding gyms in conference hotels and jogging around strange cities, as well as my own personal fitness regimen of lugging my own carry-on bags in the form of a backpack and always walking in airports —no moving sidewalks or escalators for me. I took to a series of body weight exercises in my hotel room, doing rounds of push-ups, burpees, air squats, lunges, and sit-ups. All in all, the term of my travel wasn't too bad . . . except that I got very sick.

When I started the FB50 Challenge I didn't count on a very nasty virus knocking me out of commission for nearly a month in year 1. It hit me after travelling to New Orleans for the Central Division meeting of the American Philosophical Association and then to Tucson for a workshop at the University of Arizona's Freedom Center. These were terrific and very productive research trips, but by the time I got off the plane coming home from trip two, I knew I was sick. Sore throat and cold, yes, but worst of all was a wracking cough that kept me up most nights.

Several visits to urgent care and my family doctor were the big highlights and outings in the weeks that followed. Otherwise, my exercise was limited to interval bouts of coughing and shuffling between bed and the sofa. Ugh. I was coughing so hard, I began to understand how pneumonia might kill older people.

The weeks that followed involved first working at my laptop in our comfy chair, then sitting at my desk, and then back to my standing desk.

What saw me through this setback so soon into our challenge?

First, I was relieved it happened in winter. I reminded myself of my outdoor exercising friends who pretty much give up moving in the dead of Canadian winter. I wouldn't be alone coming back after time spent in a slump.

Also, I reminded myself of my own advice to inactive beginners: Start where you are and go from there. There was no need to work out alone until I was fit enough to rejoin my communities of very fit people. And when I did go back, I checked my ego at the door of the gym, beside the rowing machine, at the edge of the mat at the dojo. I wasn't where I had been a month before, and accepting that made a difference. I reminded myself that it was supposed to be fun. I missed my physical activities. I missed my fitness friends. And I was really happy to be well enough to be back at it. Happiness outweighed the nervousness.

While I was sick I focused a lot on nutrition. When you don't feel like eating, every calorie has to count. That was a productive and useful focus. My goal was to be a better intuitive eater, as Tracy recommended, and trust my instincts more, but while sick I hadn't been eating intuitively. My inclinations were for tea, toast, and orange juice, and not much else. So it was work to keep eating protein and veggies.

Food as Fuel and Healthy Habits

Focusing on nutrition while ill was timely. I'd made a decision in the new year to try an online nutrition coaching program that promised lots of individual coaching and accountability. Their main focus was providing support for developing healthy habits.

I liked the healthy habit idea a lot. What's the difference? Rather than setting a goal—say, completing a 10K race in under an hour—you set out the steps and then commit to following the plan. Rather than picking a desired weight or percentage of body fat, you concentrate on the habits that make for healthy eating. It's simple: Make small changes, live them consistently, and change will come. That's the idea, anyway.

The two key habits the nutrition program focused on were (1) eating slowly and mindfully and (2) paying attention to hunger and eating to only 80% full. The other substantive one was eating lots of veggies and a substantial amount of protein with each meal.

They didn't rule any foods out or label some foods as "bad" or "evil." I liked that, but it meant being moderate about food choices, which tended to go against my own inclinations. I'm an all-or-nothing person. I don't smoke, I don't drink, and I don't eat meat. I started thinking about my preference for all or nothing after reading Gretchen Rubin's *The Happiness Project*. According to Rubin,

> You're a *moderator* if you...
> - find that occasional indulgence heightens your pleasure—and strengthens your resolve
> - get panicky at the thought of "never" getting or doing something
>
> You're an *abstainer* if you...
> - have trouble stopping something once you've started
> - aren't tempted by things that you've decided are off-limits

Rubin, like me, is an abstainer. She finds it easier not to eat cookies than to eat only one, but she's unhappy when she eats five. I'm a much better abstainer than a moderator—but in the second six months of our challenge I had some small successes as a moderator. Both successes involved food, an area of life where abstaining is hard. You can't just give up eating.

Success story number 1 was my moderate approach to veganism. As a vegetarian I had for years been thinking that, ethically, I ought to be a vegan. That is, the same arguments that persuaded me not to eat meat ought also, if applied consistently, to have persuaded me not to eat dairy products or eggs.

But for a variety of reasons, some involving my own food preferences but others involving the need to feed hungry, growing teenagers, I'd never been able to take that step. During the FB50 Challenge I decided I'd just do as much as I reasonably could. To a rough measure, I'd aim to eat vegan two-thirds of the time. I was inspired by a feminist philosophy colleague who had similar concerns and who'd recently taken the two-thirds vegan plunge.

And I've been successful eating vegan most, but not all, of the time. I eat free-range eggs sometimes and I use fish oil supplements. In a pinch, where other protein isn't available, I'll eat sustainable seafood. So I'm not a vegan, but my efforts, I think, are better than nothing. If you think that being a vegan is too hard, it could lead you to do nothing. Perfection is the enemy of the good, so they say.

As the philosopher Tom Hurka argued in one of his ethics columns in the *Globe and Mail,* consistency is overrated as a virtue. Better to be good two-thirds of the time than to be rotten consistently![2]

Success story number 2 was my moderate approach to desserts. I'd been tempted over the years to give up desserts entirely, but I love food as celebration too much. I love birthday cake and Pi Day. (Pi Day is celebrated around the world on March 14 or 3/14 to mark the value of pi by eating pie.) But a while ago I decided enough was enough. Not every day is dessert day. I wasn't sure if I could handle having dessert just x number of days a week, but it seems that's a plan that worked for me. I got to four days, then two, and the world hasn't ended. I was happy to be moderate about desserts.

The Waves! The Wind! Sam Takes Rowing Outside

Spring also brought some excitement in the form of moving from the rowing club's boathouse to a lake for outdoor training. And I enjoyed the prospect of spending time rowing out on the lake—as Water Rat says to Mole in *The Wind in the Willows,* "Believe me, my young friend, there is NOTHING—absolutely nothing—half so much worth doing as simply messing about in boats."

But there's another side to rowing, too, which I would also soon experience. As sportswriter John Seabrook has put it,

> Marathon runners talk about hitting "the wall" at the twenty-third mile of the race. What rowers confront isn't a wall; it's a hole—an abyss of pain, which opens up in the second minute of the race. Large needles are being driven into your thigh muscles, while your forearms seem to be splitting. Then the

pain becomes confused and disorganized, not like the winded-ness of the runner or the leg burn of the biker but an all-over, savage unpleasantness. As you pass the five-hundred-meter mark, with three-quarters of the race still to row, you realize with dread that you are not going to make it to the finish, but at the same time the idea of letting your teammates down by not rowing your hardest is unthinkable. Therefore, you are going to die.[3]

Once the masters women left the clubhouse and the safety of the rowing machines and the indoor training tanks and headed out into the lake, I started to see what he meant. For me a key part of the FB50 Challenge involved taking up a new fitness activity, rowing, and that activity became decidedly more difficult in spring of the challenge's first year. It took more time than I thought it would to get comfortable out on the water. At first the boat, filled with nervous newbies, shook a bit. Getting in and out of the rowing shell was probably the most demanding part. Well, that and not tipping.

I learned that every bit of rowing is tricky, technical, and com-plicated, from getting the boat off the rack and into the water to docking and getting out gracefully when we were done.

When we first started rowing on a local lake, cold-water safety rules applied and the coach boat had to stay very close by. On rough, windy days we stayed inside and kept working on row-ing fitness on the erg or on technique in the tank. We were all equipped with safety whistles as you can't wear flotation vests while rowing. I spent a lot of time concentrating hard on not tip-ping, mostly by following the direct order, "Never let go of your oars!" (Turns out there are a lot of direct orders in rowing: "Quick hands," "Square your oars earlier," "Keep your eyes in the boat," "Go slowly up the slide," "Hard port," etc., etc.)

My group of masters women were a mixed bunch. Some had been rowing most of their adult lives, but many more were like me, either coming to rowing from another sport (like cycling) or having taken a break from rowing to raise kids. We had originally hoped to be out in an eight-person boat but it turned out to be more flexible to take out a couple of four-person boats and some doubles and singles, depending. The quad was relatively stable as these things go, though it was still the tippiest boat I've spent time in, and I've sailed small dinghies and spent time in kayaks and canoes.

What did I love about that first experience of rowing?

First was, the water! I loved being outside. But you know that. Keeping my eyes in the boat as directed did limit my appreciation of birds, fish, and flowers somewhat. It was sort of like riding a road bike as part of fast paceline—the surrounding countryside might be gorgeous, but you don't really get to look up much and notice it while riding. I focused on the arms and backs of the women in front of me, like in cycling, where I spent a lot of time looking at the backs of other peoples' bike jerseys and only see through the pack with my peripheral vision.

I also loved being part of a team. I liked the women I was rowing with, and we also had a wonderful and attentive coach who managed to yell in a way that sounds supportive. I enjoy sports best when someone else is in charge. Rowing is perfect for that, though you need to like being yelled at! Direct orders FTW. The larger club community was pretty friendly and supportive too.

Not everything was new to me, which helped. Some of the beginner lessons I'd already learned from cycling. Mistakes move backwards down the line and get amplified, for example. Going slower is harder than going fast. Rowing at a very slow pace into the dock is tricky. "Anybody can row fast," they say. Ditto slow biking races, which I've done as training drills—last to the line wins. Yay for track stands! Balance really matters. It's easier to balance on bikes and boats at speed. And in the water there's pretty direct feedback when you get something right or wrong. We would have a good stroke and all of sudden feel the boat respond. So nice! Our goal at first was simple: to increase the ratio of good to bad strokes.

It was also just fun learning something new. Making gains quickly from week to week was exciting. And London, Ontario, was a great place to learn, being home to a high-performance rowing centre. Rowing is a big deal in London, where there are high school teams and university teams as well as social rowers.

Overall, my introduction to rowing on the water was a success, but not without its challenges. Here are a few:

1. Coordination! There's no rowing at your own pace. You follow the person in the stroke seat. More than in anything else I've done—even team trials on the bike—working in time with others matters. There's no slowing down when you want to rest. You follow the person in the front of the boat, always. It doesn't matter how strong you are if your oars don't go into the water at the same time.

2. It's technically difficult, and so many different parts of the stroke matter. I was at the stage where I just got one bit right and then everything else fell apart. I was working on bending at the waist and not breaking my knees too soon, but I'd previously been working on making sure my oars were square going into the water. For the first few weeks, it turned out, I could do one or the other but not both.

3. Rowing is hard on your hands. The top of my right hand got bashed to bits because it's the left hand that crosses over the right and you want the oars at the same height. Pretty much by the end of a practice we've all nicked ourselves somewhere and have blood on our hands.

4. Keep your eyes in the boat. That's tough. But I have some experience of this with cycling—good concentration helps.

5. Port and starboard kept throwing me off after years in sailboats. What's the problem? Well, you're sitting backwards in a rowing shell, so your right hand is on port side. As a teenager I remembered learning port and starboard by thinking that *port* and *left* each have four letters, but that doesn't work when you're facing the wrong way.

6. Despite what many people think—that rowing uses your arms and back—in fact it uses many of the same muscles as cycling. You push the boat away with your legs. I have strong legs, so that's good, but riding home afterward can be a bit tiring.

I loved my summer of rowing. I loved being outside on the water. The training with other women suited me though I struggled to fit everything in: running, cycling, CrossFit, Aikido, rowing . . . I had a lot going on that spring and summer.

Burpees Hate You Too

And yet somehow I thought I'd add something else. Do you remember the burpee from elementary school gym classes? You drop to the floor and from a position like you're going to do push-ups, jump your feet forward and then jump up high. It's a simple but brutal and effective body weight exercise. As one fitness writer explains, "By combining squat thrusts with a return to standing in between each rep, the burpee is the ultimate full-body exercise. Just one seemingly simple movement challenges the muscles in your chest, arms, thighs, hamstrings, *and* abs. And because you're using your full body when doing burpees, it's one of the best exercises to burn fat."[4]

Burpees are great for all-over exercise. A CrossFit friend posted the Burpee Summer Challenge. It seemed like a good idea at the time. But it wasn't even one of those 30-day challenges. No, this was a challenge that lasted the entire summer. Starting right after the American holiday Memorial Day at the end of May, you were to do one burpee on the first day, two on the second day, and so on, until the last day when you did 101 burpees.

Keep in mind that on the day you do 101 burpees, you did 100 the day before. That didn't quite occur to me when I signed up.

I started out loving the burpee challenge. I think even up to 30 I still quite liked it. I got fast and that helped me at CrossFit. On days I showed up at CrossFit and there were burpees as part of the workout, I was so happy. I got to cross some off the list. I did burpees everywhere that summer. I did burpees as a warm-up for rowing, on the grass outside the club. I did burpees on my back deck. I was a little bit self-conscious doing burpees in public, but since I was anxious each day to cross them off my list, I got over it.

When the numbers got high enough, I started clumping the burpees into groups of 10, and then 15. I started doing burpees first thing in the morning when I got out of bed, some in the middle of the day, and the remainder of the burpees before bed.

I did eventually give in and make one concession to the burpee challenge: I didn't make up for missing days. According to the challenge, you were supposed to make up all the burpees you missed if you missed a day. I had a few days when I was sick or I'd ridden my bike too far or I was racing, and on those days I missed out on the challenge. Rather than quit, I let myself off the hook for the missing burpees. In the end I missed just six days and I felt pretty good about that. When I think back to that summer, there was a lot going on, but the thing that coloured all of the days were the burpees.

The summer of the second six months also marked my return to the world of weekend recreational racing. I did the Kincardine Women's Triathlon (in the duathlon category—run-bike-run) with Tracy and my 22-year-old daughter, Mallory. Mallory and I liked it so much that we did another event at the end the season, also a short-course triathlon and duathlon, in a provincial park where we camped for the weekend. We even won age group medals! I also took part in an adventure race, the Warrior Dash, 5 kilometres featuring many tricky obstacles, with my cousin-in-law Tara. Making exercise and racing part of my weekend summertime fun felt just right, especially when it involved friends and family.

SAM'S TYPICAL TRAINING WEEK, MARCH–AUGUST 2013

MONDAY	7 A.M. CROSSFIT; 6:30 P.M. AIKIDO
TUESDAY	6 A.M. CROSSFIT; 6 P.M. INDOOR ROWING
WEDNESDAY	7 A.M. CROSSFIT; 6:30 P.M. AIKIDO
THURSDAY	6 A.M. CROSSFIT; 6 P.M. ROWING
FRIDAY	REST DAY
SATURDAY	AIKIDO
SUNDAY	8 A.M. INDOOR ROWING

Sam's Events and Milestones, March–August 2013
- July 2013 Kincardine Women's Duathlon, Kincardine, Ontario
- July 2013 Warrior Dash, Barrie, Ontario
- July 2013 MS Bike Tour, Grand Bend, Ontario, to London, Ontario, and back, 160 km, two days
- August 2013 Chatham-Kent YMCA Duathlon, Do-a-Du distance, Duathlon, Chatham, Ontario

PART THREE

METHOD:
A How-to
for Feminist
Fitness

NINE

Hey, Girl!

The Feminization of Fitness

WAY BACK in 1880, when "cyclist" meant "male cyclist," there was lots of hand-wringing about *lady* cyclists. Today, we've got hockey and *women's* hockey, basketball and *women's* basketball. Women and their bodies have feminine ideals to uphold, and these ideals—of quiet passivity, dependence, softness, and the aversion to competition that we talked about in the last chapter—contradict the values of athleticism and sport. Recognizing this, the fitness industry does what it can to soften the edges around women's participation with all sorts of reminders of the "for women" part. The clothing options for active women scream out: "Look at me! I'm a girl!" Lots of pink. And skirts. And floral prints.

You can scout the internet for hundreds of sites with articles about looking good while you work out. If you can't get your body to match the ideal feminine shape, there are endless possibilities for investing a chunk of money in pretty workout outfits, expensive yoga pants, and the ever-popular running skirt. Who cares what your 5K time was when it's just as important to look good for the finish-line camera? Not!

We're all for making sports and fitness activities more attractive to women. If you're a woman who hasn't explored the possibilities, getting active is a fantastic way to gain confidence and a sense of your own strength and power. But there's a fine line between creating welcoming spaces where women feel comfort-able and "feminizing" them with a focus on "ladylike" values, and the message that we can (or is it *should?*) look cute or hot while we work out. If the point is to try to include women by making every-thing "feminine," or even sexy, that's a poor strategy if it makes some women feel even more excluded.

Women's-only triathlons or marathons offer a different, more supportive experience for first-timers or even long-timers. But what about themed events like "cupcake rides" and "heels on wheels" that bring women to cycling by trading on feminine ste-reotypes? That's a trickier balance.

Let's start with the colour pink.

What's So Bad about Pink Anyway?

A couple of years ago, women in the online fitness world got up in arms over a post by a popular male fitness blogger who shall remain nameless because we hate sending traffic his way. He pre-sented a list of over 100 strength-training "tips" for women. He observed that women tend to like wearing pink to the gym. He said it like a criticism. Because obviously a true athlete (read: man) would *never* gravitate toward such a girly colour.

Commenters on the post and commentators from other blogs had varied responses to the point about pink, ranging from "Sometimes it's hard to find something functional, that fits, and that *isn't* pink" to "What's so bad about pink anyway?"

The post's author admitted that he hadn't given any thought to the difference in availability of pink clothing for women and for men. He was completely bewildered one day when five of his female clients showed up with some pink on their outfits, remark-ing that none of his male clients would ever do that. As if the guys and the women had exactly the same colour palettes available to them when they went shopping for their fitness clothing.

Let's be clear about something here. What's so bad about pink has nothing to do with the colour itself. It's lovely. The trouble starts when you combine lack of choice for women with what we call the "social meaning" of pink.

In the Western world, we socialize girls into pink before birth. Prospective parents who know "it's a girl!" have the go-ahead to start decorating the nursery in pink, buying pink clothes for the baby, and stocking up on pink accessories. When the baby is born, into a pink blanket she goes.

Have you ever asked for clothes in gender-neutral colours like green and orange and purple when shopping for duds for kids? If you want the salesperson to look at you as if you have three heads, try it. Without pink, how we would ever be able to tell the girls' stuff from the boys' stuff? Pink stands as a powerful, consistent, and virtually inescapable marker of all things feminine. Enter the girls' clothing department or even the girls' part of a toy shop and you will find yourself in a sea of pink.

It's not much different for women seeking workout clothes. Yes, there are some choices sometimes. But if you look carefully, you will see that there is a heck of a lot of pink—neon pink, baby pink, antique pink, rosy pink... You'll see it on shoelaces, soles, and trim. It's the feature colour for yoga tops, running tops, jackets, even socks and accessories like water bottles, hats, and headbands. We own pink stuff, and you probably do too. We like our pink things (and you probably do too). Why? Not because of our chromosomes, that's for sure! Because of a complicated mix of what we may have been conditioned to like and what's available.

So what's the *social meaning* of pink? It's all about "feminine"—girlish, dependent, a little bit silly, a little bit soft, a little bit fickle, cute, and just generally weak. Of course, that doesn't mean girls and women are actually this way. Not at all. But femininity as a cultural ideal likes to represent us this way. Add a bit of zip to the pink, going for neon instead of pastel, and you've got sexy, too.

Pink's association with femininity means that when men dare choose to wear pink, they "must be gay." If a boy likes and wears pink to school, he risks ridicule and bullying.

But wait. What about the thoroughly macho, straight man in a position of power who wears pink? In those cases pink has the paradoxically opposite effect of making people even more enthralled by his masculinity. He's *so* masculine he can wear pink without having his sexuality called into question.

It doesn't end with pink workout wear. You can get pink equipment: dumbbells, kettlebells, stability balls, BOSUs, foam rollers... But lots of us lift weights to get *strong*, and the stereotypical associations with pink just aren't all that empowering. Not to mention that the high end for pink dumbbells is usually about five pounds, with two and three pounds being more common. No one is going to get all that strong lifting only pink weights.

We don't want to be the pink police. If you want to wear pink, if you want to look cute in the gym, then you have a right to do that. But in the social context we live in, pink doesn't do us any favours in the gym. And if you consider the many pink items available to women and not to men, we have to wonder how much choice there really is.

As feminist scholars, both of us reflect on the way social forces shape women's choices and preferences. Face it: it's not some biologically innate feature of girls and women that we like pink stuff. It's not in our DNA. Pink is just a colour. That's why it may seem innocuous, but its social meaning can take away our power in certain contexts. And at the moment, the gym is one of those contexts.

Changing entrenched social meanings doesn't happen overnight. And it doesn't happen without an awareness of the pernicious messages about women and femininity. As women, when we choose to wear pink, it's good to be aware that we are choosing more than a colour, and that our desires, preferences, and options have been heavily influenced by our upbringing and environment.

Sometimes that awareness alone might prompt us to question our choices long enough to ask, "Is this available in another colour?" And when we do ask that, wouldn't it be great if at least some of the time the answer to that question could be "Yes"?

Play Hard, Look Cute

Pink is not the alpha and the omega of the feminization of sport and fitness. The "play hard, look cute" mentality extends far beyond the colour palette of workout clothing and gear.

Every January the *Huffington Post* publishes something about how motivating cute workout gear can be in getting us to the gym. In 2013 it was "Cute Workout Clothes Are the Key to Getting You Off the Couch and to the Gym (PHOTOS)." The photos are before-and-after workout gear makeovers. In 2015, it was "Cute Workout Clothes That Will Actually Make You Want to Hit the Gym. Seriously." There, the photos focus on fashionable ensembles for a host of activities from Pilates to kick-boxing.

And what about running skirts? Or the difference between men's beach volleyball uniforms—long shorts and tank tops, similar to what you see on the basketball court—and women's beach volleyball uniforms—skimpy bikini bottoms and sports bras. We're talking about world-class competitors in the Olympics.

But what's the problem? All too often women are sexualized in sport, not taken seriously. Athleticism takes a back seat to sex appeal. It reinforces the idea that even when women are athletes, they need to look a certain way. Attractiveness to straight men is the filter through which all must pass. Have you ever had that feeling that you have to pass muster on this score before you're welcome in the gym or on the court or track?

The feminization of sports sends one specific message: Women are lesser athletes than men. Men's sports are the real sports; women's are the poor cousin. Aesthetics first, athletic accomplishment second. It's a way of downplaying women's potential, giving us something else that we need to be obsessed about, something besides how we play, lift, run, pass, kick, skate, hit, swim, bike, or jump. And if women's sports are lesser, then we will see less funding going into them. We will see fewer women getting out there and learning to use their bodies in powerful and skilful ways.

Research shows that one of the key reasons women avoid the gym or feel discouraged before they get there is that they are uncomfortable being seen in the clothing that we've come to associate with working out. Form-fitting shorts and tights, sports bras, and revealing exercise-wear has turned many a woman off before she even gets started. Sure, you can always choose not to wear that. But a gym is an intimidating environment already, and for some, having the right "uniform" is a way of fitting in. If you're already feeling out of place, then that's just one more way of emphasizing that you don't really belong. To be sure, this is about body image as much as it is about fashion. But sports fashion is not only aesthetic. It's also about performance-oriented styles. You can't do a time trial in baggy sweatpants and a hoodie.

If you're nervous about putting yourself out there, there are ways of getting past it. Awareness and knowledge can both go a long way. Tracy's past experience taught her that feeling comfortable in a space makes a huge difference to how likely she is to go there. And a lot of that comfort comes from knowing how to use the equipment properly. If you can walk around like you own the place and know exactly what you are doing and where you are going next, that gives you a lot of gym cred.

But by the time we embarked on the FB50 Challenge, Tracy had been out of the weight room for over a decade. She'd lost that feeling of confidence based on solid knowledge of what to do. In the intervening years, some of the equipment had changed, and again, there seemed to be the things the guys did (free weights) and the things the women did (routines with stability balls). No longer a graduate student, she didn't belong to the dominant demographic in the gym anymore—young, fit, and strong. One dimension of the feminization of fitness is that lots of people assume that women, especially older women, don't know how to use the equipment. The psychological impact of knowing that people assume you don't know what you're doing can affect performance. It exacerbates the feeling of awkwardness and not belonging. It makes a person more likely to fumble. It also makes it harder to ask for help: even though Tracy actually knew how to use most of the equipment, when it came to something she didn't know how to use, she felt hesitant to ask for fear of playing into the stereotype that she, an older woman, had no idea what she was doing.

Tracy's quite a confident woman with a long history of weight training in a mixed-gender environment. If being new in a gym can affect her that way, then just imagine how it is for less experienced women, women who are perceived to be overweight, older women, or any women who do not fit the normative expectations we impose on people who use gyms. Remember, there are women using treadmills in sheds so as not to be seen and judged, for goodness' sake! It's just sad. But we can challenge that stuff.

With our FB50 Challenge underway, it took Tracy at least a year to work her way back to feeling totally at home in the gym. The comfort came from consciously not falling into line with a gendered approach to workouts. No pink weights and fluffy kettlebells for her.

Women-Only Events and Spaces

A mutual friend of ours once said she didn't believe in shaving her legs, but she had an even more difficult time when standing in line at the ATM thinking people were staring at her hairy legs and judging her, so she shaved her legs. Your workouts might be like that for you—you're just not up to making a feminist statement in that area of your life, not up to the internal battle required to claim that space as yours.

One way around this feeling of not fitting in is to join a women's-only gym or enter women's-only events. We've both tried women-only events and always have a great time. They do have a different vibe than the mixed-gender events, and we think they're great starting points for new athletes. For both of us, the Kincardine Women's Triathlon was our first. The event fills up quickly, which is a testament to its popularity with return competitors and to the good press it gets as a fun race for new women triathletes to sharpen their teeth on.

You can find women's half marathons, like the Niagara Falls Women's Half Marathon—a favourite among Tracy's running circle—and women's run series, like the Toronto Women's Run Series. The Dirty Girl event is the women-only version of the Tough Mudder, if you want to try one of those obstacle-challenge races gaining traction these days as the new fun thing.

Some people charge women-only events with sexism because, well, they exclude half the human race. Feminists are used to this kind of challenge, which is often made to the idea of women-only spaces. We object to men's clubs and things like that, so why is it okay to exclude men when the roles are reversed? How would we feel about men-only events? The Boston Marathon was deemed sexist when it used to exclude women. That's why Kathy Switzer, the first women to run it, counts as a pioneer in women's sport. Yet she's a great supporter of the annual Niagara Women's Half Marathon. (Aside: the Niagara Women's Half doesn't actually exclude men, but men's results don't qualify them for prizes in their age groups or overall, and the T-shirts aren't sized with them in mind.) Why are these sorts of events suspect when they're reserved for men but causes for celebration when reserved for women? Another worry about women-only events is that they exclude gender non-conforming athletes, that is, athletes who don't fit comfortably on the gender binary. People who don't sit on either side on the gender binary aren't so well served by men's and women's separate events or by men's and women's combined events where athletes must tick off a box. Gender non-conforming athletes may prefer that events not be sorted by sex at all. So women-only events won't solve all the problems of gender inclusion in sports.

Women-only and girls-only spaces make sense if you believe, as we do, that girls and women have been structurally and systemically disadvantaged by a society that implicitly privileges men. That means men have all sorts of advantages that pass for normal: they hold more positions of power, people take them more seriously, they earn more money, and the list goes on. This type of structural advantage doesn't only come to men—there's also white privilege, class privilege, non-disabled privilege, heterosexual privilege . . . But gender is a biggie. Opportunities for women as members of a systemically disadvantaged group do not make men worse off. Why not? Because men already enjoy social privilege and entitlement in all sorts of public arenas, including sports.

Why is an event with only women attractive to women? This question has more than one answer.

One of the main reasons is that a women-only environment feels more like a "safe space" for taking risks. Research shows that we see fewer women in sports from CrossFit to triathlon. Certain areas of the gym, such as the weight room, tend to attract fewer women. As philosophers, we both like to press these facts and ask, "Why?" For many women, it's a confidence issue. It's hard enough to put yourself out there—harder still in a mixed-gender environment. And it's not just because we're worrying about our skills and abilities. There are also insecurities about how we might look when working out (remember the sheds!). Women-only spaces like women's gyms can minimize these impediments. They also relieve some of the perceived pressures to conform to the feminine appearance norms. Other arguments for women-only gyms or sections of gyms have to do with perceived differences in gym etiquette between men and women. When the downtown YMCA in Vancouver moved to close its women-only section, some women objected on the grounds that they had a right to space where they would not be "watched, cat-called, or have their form corrected by a man." Others talked about the discomfort working alongside grunting men who didn't clean their sweat off of the equipment (not that all men grunt and walk away from dirty equipment, of course).[1]

The gym was phasing out its women-only section because, they said, it was underused. But one reason it was underused is that it did not have the same range of equipment available in the mixed section. Women-only spaces are great for all the reasons we've outlined, but let's not shortchange women by having their spaces be inferior. If we want to enable women to thrive, then simply segregating them with poor facilities is not acceptable. Assuming that a women's gym is adequately equipped, it can offer a positive alternative for women who might otherwise feel uncomfortable working out in a gym.

Does the idea that women might thrive more easily in scenarios where men are taken out of the equation translate to the women-only racing events? The founder of the Kincardine Women's Triathlon says her event gives women a race where they can feel empowered and comfortable. Other women-only triathlons promote the idea of "racing with your friends" and "celebrating women's sport with the beginner in mind." It's less about competition and more about solidarity.

Some organized activities for women, such as the Cupcake Ride and Heels on Wheels, have a different angle on attracting women. The Cupcake Rides in Toronto are the brainchildren of Hyedie Hashimoto, who had made it her mission to get girls and women out on bikes. These women-only rides begin and end at bakeries (hence "the Cupcake Ride"). Heels on Wheels is a little bit different. It's a group ride, also for women, but lots of them wear high heels. You can also find Belles on Bikes, a similar event that plays up femininity while promoting cycling.

These types of events and groups associate women on bikes with femininity rather than athleticism. Maybe you think, sure, if that's what gets women out on bikes, then so be it. Lure us in with cupcakes and high heels. We'll be downing sport gels, talking bike components, comparing our bike computers, and donning high-end race kits in no time. Possibly. It's true that lots of women care about their femininity and avoid physically demanding activities for fear of coming across as unfeminine. If we can combine femininity and activity, that may open things up for some women. At the same time, we worry about perpetuating the idea of "activity lite" for women and leaving the real physically challenging stuff for men. And like we said before, lots of women don't like pink, never wear heels, and might never eat a cupcake. Gender stereotyping isn't always inclusive.

The Niagara Falls Women's Half Marathon tries to strike a balance. It appeals to some of the preferences we attribute to women—wine and cosmetics in the swag bag, flowers and lavender in all the temporary toilets, firefighters in charge of the finishers' medals. They pitch it as a fun weekend getaway to Niagara with "your girlfriends" and an "empowering celebration of health and fitness." At the same time, it's a half marathon—hardly a trivial distance—so it can't be all daisies and fizzy lemonade.

The women's triathlons that position themselves as fun events where women can feel empowered and comfortable don't include pink cupcakes and high heels. In this respect, they focus on triathlon as sport. Nevertheless, they downplay the competitive aspect. The Race for Life (a run to fundraise for cancer research) in the UK has a page on its website that addresses the "women only" issue for its event:

> We regularly review our events to make them the best they can be. Two years ago, we seriously investigated the possibility of including men in Race for Life. However, our research shows that a significant number of our Race for Life supporters would strongly prefer to keep it a female-only event as it is a unique opportunity for women to come together in a non-competitive environment within an atmosphere of 'sisterhood'.[2]

But women are all different and have their own levels of confidence and athleticism. Sam likes funky shoes and jewellery, even has skirts, dresses, and pink stuff in her wardrobe. But when she goes out for a run she doesn't wash her hair first. Instead, she splashes cold water on her face and flings a hat on over messy hair. She does the same for cycling with her helmet. She leaves the girly stuff behind when she's doing sporty things because the norms of ladylike behaviour pull against the norms of sports performance. It's not just that trying to look cute means there's less energy for thinking about winning. It's more than that.

Sam has worn a rowing unisuit that was probably the least flattering piece of clothing there is and a racing swimsuit that was tight and didn't leave much to the imagination. But in both cases the point is speed, not looks. Her male cyclist friends had to teach her how to spit and blow her nose from the bike (hint: you don't use a tissue!). She had to overcome an aversion to hitting and punching others so she could advance in Aikido. In all of these activities, adhering to norms of femininity would have meant sacrificing performance.

Women-only events are a great middle ground between acknowledging, on the one hand, that women are also entitled to engage in these activities and, on the other, that for many women these are new pursuits that might feel intimidating. Participating with women only helps to take the edge off just a little. And since few of us have fully escaped our socialization into at least some feminine qualities, these sorts of events can be supportive and empowering. That makes them more fun and less stressful.

It's even gotten Tracy to wonder sometimes whether she loves triathlon or just the Kincardine Women's Triathlon! (She loves both.)

Take it away...

One size doesn't fit all. Including women takes more than "shrinking it and pinking it," as they say in retail. Women aren't just smaller, cuter men! Women-only spaces and events have a lot going for them, as long as they don't make assumptions about women's needs and wants based on outdated stereotypes about women as "the weaker sex."

Try this...

There are lots of different ways to be a woman in sports. Find out what works for you. Maybe you want to work out in a women-only space or try a women-only event. Go for it! Or if you would rather mix it up with the guys on the soccer field or volleyball court, join a league! Figure out which types of gendered (or non-gendered) spaces work for you.

TEN

Exercise in Everyday Life

HOW DOES exercise fit into your life? Do you schedule it or do you wear a tracking device that counts all the movements in your day?

If physical activity in your life always involves special clothes and driving someplace to start and the activity has a sharp beginning and end time, then when it comes to exercise, you're a compartmentalizer. You think of exercise as a *special* sort of thing that you do. Maybe you call it "working out." Sam has a friend who defends driving to the gym and taking the elevator to the weight room because he jokes that he likes to arrive "fresh" for his workout. He's definitely a compartmentalizer. He does no exercise unless it's a prescribed workout at the gym.

Integrationists, on the other hand, try to work physical activity into the fabric of their everyday lives. We're always exercising, whether walking to work, standing and talking to other people, carrying groceries into the house, doing laundry, mowing lawns, or running errands on foot—you get the idea. No special clothes required.

Our modern lives can be incredibly sedentary, and even physically fit people can spend far too much time sitting. Most people seem to focus on compartmentalized exercise—like going to the gym or getting out for a run—but it looks like we need to add more movement back into our everyday lives, where possible, when possible, if we're really going to get fit. Settle in for some alarming research on human movement and how much we've slowed down.

Engineering Movement Out of Our Lives

Our modern lives require us to move an astonishingly tiny amount. It's as if, for those of us in middle class of the Western world, we've engineered it all away. We drive to work. We sit at our desks all day. We sit down for meals, often meals that we haven't even prepared ourselves. Even housework takes less effort than it once did. Oodles of different devices make our lives easier, from dishwashers to drive-through banks. Modern houses have a second-storey laundry room so you don't need to walk up and down the stairs carrying hampers and baskets of clothes and sheets. Very few people use clotheslines or push mowers. More and more houses come with built-in elevators. Think about the advances that come with a cost in terms of strength and movement. We all love automatic garage door openers and television remote controls, but now we're no longer using our muscles to open the garage door or taking those few extra steps when we want to change channels. There's automatic everything! In our childhoods we had to manually crank down car windows, but no more. It happens at work too. We don't even have to walk down the hall to ask a colleague a question—email is easier.

On the one hand, it's great that everything is easier. People with physical challenges and limits have seen huge gains. Older people can stay in their own homes for longer. But as with moving sidewalks in airports—meant for those who can't easily cover long distances with baggage—these options make it easier for *everyone* to move less.

How much less are we moving? A lot less. And it's bad. Our bodies are made to move. According to a 2014 study by the Physical Activity Council, more than a quarter of the U.S. population—28%—did not participate in a single physical activity the previous year. The physical activity as the study defined it didn't have to be something super-intense like mixed martial arts or quarterbacking for the New York Jets. Stretching was considered an activity. The number of Americans who could be described as "totally sedentary" has risen to its highest level since 2007. Things might be a bit better in Canada, but not very much. According to Statistics Canada's 2011 Canadian Health Measures Survey, only 15% of adults achieve the minimum amount of daily recommended exercise.

The focus on exercise leaves out the range of everyday movement that is part of our lives. Lying down in bed is worse from a movement point of view than sitting, sitting is worse than standing, and standing is worse than walking—even walking around the house. We've also become critical of fidgeting and restless movement, but even fidgeting is useful from the perspective of total activity.

And non-exercise physical activity makes a huge difference. People who stand more than three hours a day live around three years longer than their more sedentary peers. "Sitting for extended periods of time has been linked with heart disease, diabetes, cancer and obesity," says the National Academy of Sports Medicine's April Plank. "Getting up hourly and walking to the restroom, getting a refill of water or standing up to stretch can decrease stiffness, boost energy and burn calories. Also, when watching TV, during every commercial break get up and move. Do a few stretches, walk around the house or bust out a few bicep curls."[1] Lots of our academic friends set timers for writing in blocks of time and use the end of the block as a reminder to move, say, 25 minutes of writing and 5 minutes of movement.

The Dangers of Sitting

The aspect of "not moving" that's got the most attention in the past few years is sitting. You'd have to be living under a rock not to have read something about the dangers of sitting. Experts have taken to talking about "sedentary disease." The list of ill-health effects associated with sitting includes heart disease, diabetes, cancer, and other conditions that occur as your muscles switch into a "dormant" mode that compromises their ability to break down fats and sugars. Exercising before or after work isn't enough to counteract these effects—sitting all day is harmful no matter how fit and active you are.

In fact, occupational sitting time is where the epidemiology of physical activity first began. In the 1950s, Jeremy Morris found that London's double-decker bus drivers were more likely to die from cardiovascular disease than were bus conductors, and that government clerks were more likely to die than mail carriers.[2] In both cases, the more sedentary job carried greater health risks than the more active job, even though they were in a similar line of work. In the decades that followed, researchers and policy makers focused on the health benefits of getting exercise. But according to the latest research, even when people do significant and regular exercise, they still increase their risks of serious illness from hours of physical inactivity. These findings are also consistent with lifestyles in Blue Zones, places such as Okinawa, Japan, and Sardinia, Italy, where people live much longer on average than the rest of the developed world. In addition to plant-based diets and strong communities, near-constant moderate physical activity is the norm in these areas.

But not everyone can stand or get up and walk around. Many people spend the day in wheelchairs. "Just Stand," the slogan of a company that makes standing desks, assumes that standing is an option. Many health campaigns make this mistake too, such as those that focus on taking the stairs instead of the elevator. Again, not everyone can do that. Some of us have back problems that mean we can't sit all day. Others have bodies that can't stand. Human bodies and abilities vary.

In her class on sports ethics, Sam uses a wonderful documentary called *FIXED: The Science/Fiction of Human Enhancement*. The film's description reads: "From bionic limbs and neural implants to prenatal screening, researchers around the world are hard at work developing a myriad of technologies to fix or enhance the human body. *FIXED: The Science/Fiction of Human Enhancement* takes a close look at the drive to be 'better than human' and the radical technological innovations that may take us there." One of the most interesting characters in the documentary is Gregor Wolbring, a professor at the University of Calgary. It's striking to watch Wolbring crawl around his home—his preferred mode of mobility. But crawling makes people who can walk squeamish. In one scene Wolbring boards a plane by crawling up the steps and down the aisle, and the flight attendants seem uncomfortable. Or maybe it's the viewer, you and me, that it makes uncomfortable. When writing this chapter, we even wondered whether there might a word other than *crawling* to describe the way Wolbring moves. Why? Because we associate crawling with a lack of dignity.

But Wolbring looks speedy and agile on the ground, getting in and out of his car, and boarding a plane crawling up the steps and down the aisle to his seat. His graceful, speedy movement challenges our stereotypes of what the human body can do. By comparison, the wheelchair is normalizing in the sense that non-disabled people aren't made uncomfortable by it. The non-disabled are more comfortable with people in chairs than with people using alternative modes of bodily movement.

The link between disability and being sedentary also works the other way. Being sedentary makes it more likely that you'll become disabled. Researchers are finding that sedentary behaviours like sitting just an hour extra per day can up your risk for disabilities in later life—even if you are otherwise moderately active.[3]

As academics, we both sit a lot at work, and not just at our desks. We also attend academic conferences and travel by air to get to them. While writing this chapter, Sam flew to California twice in one month—five hours of sitting in each direction. On her way home, her seatmate, a cancer researcher travelling to an academic conference, said the research he read had convinced him. In flight, he followed his usual practice. He set his alarm and got up every 20 minutes. With the permission of the flight attendants, he stood at the back of the plane. But every passenger can't do that—there just isn't room.

And then, once you're off the plane, there's the conference itself. If the regular working day is a 5K or 10K run, conferences are sitting marathons. At one conference Sam attended, sessions started at 9 a.m. and ended at 9 p.m. with very few breaks. Most sessions came in three-hour chunks, sometimes without any time out to stand or walk during them. And then there's teaching. The professor gets to stand and walk, but what about our students? Sam tries to get people up at least once in a one-hour lecture. It's easy to get lots of movement in your day if you're a mail carrier but much less easy if you drive a truck or a city bus for living. Most administrative jobs that involve sitting in cubicles can be challenging: if you stand to talk on the phone or get up and walk around, you disturb others. But many people have jobs that involve a lot of sedentary time, and finding ways to break it up can limit the negative effects on our health.

Some people respond to concerns about sitting with skepticism about so-called all-cause mortality. The all-cause mortality rate is the number of people who die in a given age group of any and all causes. Why is all-cause mortality not the best measure? Research in medicine often uses mortality as an important outcome. Death is easy to measure, it's not subject to misclassification, and it's the most important outcome for many conditions and treatments. But we all have to die of something, and all-cause mortality just points to a correlation without a specific disease story about how sitting hurts us.

However, sitting isn't just tied to higher all-cause mortality. It's been linked to some very specific diseases and conditions, such as a heightened risk of cancer, specifically lung cancer, colon, and endometrial cancer. Sitting time was not related to other cancers, however, including breast, rectal, ovarian, prostate, esophageal, or testicular cancers.

You might think that young people do better on the not sitting front—oh, that we could all be as active as in our youth! But you'd be wrong. According to researchers at the University of Limerick, young women sit or lie down for an alarming portion of the day. The 2011 study found that teenage girls lie or sit for up to 19 hours a day, including long bouts of inactivity during school. The researchers suggested that although the girls might be getting enough exercise, "if you sit for the rest of the day, it will still have health consequences." "There is no doubt that performing moderate or vigorous physical activity is good for the long term health of adolescents," Alan Donnelly says. However, he believes that "long periods of sitting might be a separate risk factor in this group."[4]

Can you undo the ill-health effects of sitting, or if you've already been sitting your whole career, are you basically doomed?

There *are* some things you can start doing now. First, and most obvious, spend less time sitting. The Booker Prize–nominated writer Emma Donoghue (author of *Room*) calls her treadmill desk "a miracle." Less drastic measures include getting up and stretching every 20 minutes. Researchers say that that undoes a lot of the ill effects of sitting. It's not just total time that matters: it seems to matter most how long you sit at a time without a break. Some workplaces have taken to having standing or walking meetings. Apparently, these are even shorter and more productive. You can also exercise at work, and, of course, since television invites sitting, watch less television. We also need to move beyond thinking about this as an individual problem and think about big-picture workplace situations. Many people have jobs where they don't have control over how much they sit or the hours they work.

Sedentary Athletes

Now, you might think the dangers of not moving during the day matters only to those people who don't also exercise. But no. Heavy exercisers, it turns out, often move *less* the rest of the day and so burn not that many more calories than if they hadn't exercised at all. When not exercising, many athletes are chronic sitters. "Even competitive athletes who do double workouts often live a sedentary lifestyle," says sports nutritionist Nancy Clark. "They generally do little but rest and recover during the non-exercise parts of their day."[5]

Gretchen Reynolds has written about the study that set out to prove this, both in *The First 20 Minutes* and in her popular *New York Times* Phys Ed blog. The University of Copenhagen study followed a group of young men assigned to a heavy exercise program, but found that they lost little weight. Yes, they ate more, but more surprisingly, "they also were resolutely inactive in the hours outside of exercise, the motion sensors show[ed]. When they weren't working out, they were, for the most part, sitting. 'I think they were fatigued,'" concluded researcher Mads Rosenkilde.[6]

While we're not professional athletes, it's true for many like us that the primary movement we get in a day is our purposeful workout or training session.

Are Chairs Evil?

So far the talk about the dangers of sitting, whether among sedentary athletes or university professors, has looked at the issue as (mostly) a matter of individual choice. But it's also a matter of institutional design. We sit in chairs because chairs are provided. If we have them in our houses, it's because it's furniture we're expected to buy for our homes.

According to author Colin McSwiggen, who wrote a piece called "Against Chairs," recent writing about the problem of sitting describes the situation in ways that mislead. It gets the focus wrong when it looks at individual choice. He writes, "They make it look like the problem is just that we sit too much. The real problem is that sitting, in our society, usually means putting your body in a raised seat with back support—a chair. Sitting wouldn't be so bad if we didn't sit on things that are bad for us."[7] Modern chairs are evil, says McSwiggen.

But, you might wonder, what's new about this? Weren't there always chairs? How are we just learning now that they're bad?

First, chairs aren't universal. In lots of places people engage in what ergonomics experts call *active sitting*. Active sitting postures include squatting and sitting cross-legged. They're a bit like chair sitting but they aren't bad for you the way chair sitting is. Second, according to McSwiggen's fascinating history of the chair, chairs are also relatively new. He dates the mass adoption of chairs to the Industrial Revolution.

Third, you might be tempted to think that the answer lies in a better chair. But it's not clear what a good chair would even be. You've all seen the many variations: the kneeling chair, the stability ball as chair, the wobbly stool as chair, to list just some. But what should a good chair do? A good chair should encourage you to leave it at frequent intervals, not settle in for the day (and night). That lumpy lounger that no one wants to sit in or the hard-as-rock dining chair you haul out when extra guests arrive? Perfect.

Doing research for the blog and for this book, Sam started to realize just how much sitting she did. As a writer, an academic, and, for a time, an administrator, she sat for most of the day. Though she's never watched a lot of television, she reads a lot in the evening, usually sitting in her comfy reading chair, the same chair where she often sits and grades undergraduate essays and where she sat for years nursing infants and reading to toddlers. It's a chair with both "professor" and "mom" associations.

Sitting at work didn't come naturally, says Sam. She's a fidgeter by temperament and usually a restless pacer. Once she discovered exercise, she thought she'd found the solution: run, lift, ride into physical exhaustion, shower, eat, and then write. Physically exhausted but mentally alert was her best state for getting academic tasks completed. She wrote good chunks of her dissertation that way and had a fantastically productive sabbatical training with a cycling club at 6 a.m. and arriving at her office desk, with body worn out, mind ready to go, by nine. She'd been pretty certain that the amount of exercise she did trumped the amount of time she spent sitting.

Sam learned she was wrong from reading A. J. Jacobs's *Drop Dead Healthy,* in which he chronicles the year in which he tried a different piece of health advice each month. Standing (or walking) to write is one of the recommendations Jacobs keeps after his year. Sam was intrigued. Coincidentally, the concern about sitting as a health risk corresponded for her to nagging back pain. When a physiotherapist said Sam had excellent standing posture but really needed to work on her sitting posture, she was annoyed. She left her office strapped up with postural taping—the sort that doesn't hold you in place but makes you realize if you're slumping—and a keen desire to find another solution.

As she started looking at the literature on workplace ergonomics, she kept returning to the pictures of standing desks. A light bulb went on. "How about a standing desk?" "That would be terrific. Are you willing to give it a try?" Yes!

Sam was about to begin her first at-home sabbatical, six months free from teaching and administration to focus on her own academic projects. A typical sabbatical workload of 90% research and writing usually means lots of time sitting. The timing was right to give the standing desk a try. She switched at first to a make-it-yourself standing desk at home. She followed the instructions on one of the many "how to make your standing desk out of readily available materials" websites and loved it. Others go the DIY route to make their own treadmill desks. You don't need a good treadmill, with fancy controls and bells and whistles. After all, you're not going to run on it. You're just going to turn it into a desk you can walk at, so you can buy one of the many treadmills for sale in thrift stores or in classifieds online.

Sam enjoyed her standing desk right from the start and felt more alive, engaged, and on task when writing while standing. The desk itself was pretty much free, though she did purchase a shock-absorbing floor mat, the kind used by chefs on stone floors, or cashiers who work long shifts on their feet.

Her family's reaction to the standing desk was amusing. Sam's parents live next door and come and go often. They'd both had long careers in physically demanding jobs, as bakers, and the idea of standing when you don't have to seemed strange to them.

At the end of the first year of our FB50 Challenge, in September 2013, Sam switched to a height-adjustable desk at work and now spends about half of the day on her feet. The university quit paying for back physio and instead bought her the fancy desk.

Besides the energy and feeling of being alive and on task that comes with standing, Sam thinks it makes her write better. Posture matters and standing makes her feel engaged and in touch with the ground. She also quit endless, pointless web surfing. Over the years she's started standing in meetings too, and at university lectures. She's also been asking her graduate students to walk and talk about their latest chapter. They go along with it cheerfully. It helps that she's the supervisor.

By the end of the FB50 Challenge, Sam had even taken to eating while standing, against decades of diet advice. The standard advice—*Thou shalt not eat while standing*—is practically one of the Ten Commandments of dieting. Eat at the table. Make an occasion of it. Don't read or watch television. Pay attention to your food. The no-standing rule is one of the few adhered to and recommended by our extreme dieting culture and even by those who advocate intuitive eating. Do you know this rule? For better or worse, it's false.

The theory is that you're more likely to enjoy your food and pace yourself if you're sitting down. Surely, speed of eating is an independent variable, not necessarily tied to whether you sit or stand? Now the Livestrong fitness website has taken one step forward, recommending that we aim to eat one meal a day while standing. They suggest trying this at breakfast, standing at the kitchen counter, or having lunch at a place with tall tables.[8]

Sam is on board for this advice. She's been savouring dinner on her feet in the kitchen when eating alone. She sets a place at the kitchen counter, and loves it.

Driving Ourselves into the Grave?

If sitting is one bad thing we do lots of, driving is another. Changing that routine is also an excellent way to work some everyday exercise into your life. At our workplace, a university campus, different groups vie for access to the closest parking. But why? Why don't we walk more? Recent research shows that even people who use the bus or other forms of public transport get a lot more movement in than those who drive to and from work. They have not only better overall fitness as a result but also lower blood pressure and lower rates of obesity.[9] That surprised us. We knew that walking or biking beat out driving, but taking the bus? What's the explanation? It turns out that the walking we do to get to and from bus stops makes a pretty big difference over time. The message? It all adds up.

The rise and ubiquity of smartphones and fitness trackers means that we now have lots of data to back up claims we always thought were true. Just as public transit users walk more than those who drive or get driven, so too do urban dwellers walk a lot more than those who dwell in the suburbs. They walk about twice as much, in fact.[10]

There are also big differences between countries. The average Australian walks about 9,500 steps a day, Americans just half that.[11] Is there something magical about the 10,000 number when it comes to steps? Perhaps not, but 5,000 is very little movement. Interestingly, Canadians fall in the middle. We don't do as well as the Australians, but we're not as sedentary as our American neighbours.

The idea of incorporating exercise into our everyday lives has always had an appeal for us. In the early days of her career, Tracy had an apartment close enough to the university that she could walk, far enough that it was "a good walk." But by the time the FB50 Challenge came along about 20 years later, walking to work was occasional at best for her. Tracy had slipped into the habit of driving every day.

So what happened? Driving just seemed more convenient. It allowed her to seamlessly incorporate errands into her commute, and she could just toss her yoga gear into the back of the car and make it to a class at the end of the workday without having to go home first. You know how it is. Busy woman, full life, and so it went.

The first year of FB50, Tracy eased into it on one of the blessings of academic life: study leave. It felt easy to give up the parking pass that year.

Switching up the walking with some cycling posed a bigger challenge. Tracy made herself more comfortable by treating herself to a new bicycle for her 48th birthday, a sturdy hybrid with easy shifting, disc brakes, fenders so she wouldn't arrive at work with a line of mud up her back, and a rear rack that she could snap her cool new pannier to.

The real test of Tracy's resolve came when her study leave ended, one year into the challenge and just before her 49th birthday. She didn't renew the parking permit. Instead, she tuned up the commuter bike and got used to riding it with the pannier cram-jammed with books and laptop and lunch. She rode into the late summer and fall. To make it manageable, she allowed herself two strips of bus tickets a month (that's 10 rides and $19). Being kinder to herself and the environment saved her money and lowered her stress level—turned out all that rushing around cramming in errands on either side of the workday had had nothing going for it besides convenience.

So while Sam hacked her workday routine, opting for a standing desk, Tracy hacked her commute. What do *you* do to get some everyday exercise into your life?

Take it away...
When it comes to exercise, are you a compartmentalizer or an integrationist? Whichever you are, it's not a bad idea to think about ways to integrate exercise into your daily routine. We are more sedentary today than people were a few decades ago, and the research shows that sitting decreases our lifespan.

Try this...

If you have a desk job, try a standing desk or even a treadmill desk, or get up periodically. Walk or bike to work. There are lots of ways to get active in our everyday lives, even for those who are compartmentalizers at heart.

ELEVEN
Let's Move!
Taking Care of Our Cardio Health

IF YOU'VE ever embarked on a fitness program, you've heard of cardio. We like to think of it as a form of cross-training, because it's a good thing to include as one part of a fitness program. Love it or hate it, you can't make any claims to true fitness without cardio. Cardio fitness—or cardiovascular fitness, as it's more properly called—is the ability of your heart and lungs to pump oxygen rich blood to your muscles so that you can move. "Cardio" is also the name for the kind of exercise that gets you out of breath and makes your heart pound. When you do cardio, you're training your heart as a muscle and making it stronger.

Maybe you have your cardio favourites—Sam has a passion for cycling, for Tracy it's a toss-up between running and swimming. No one doubts that a good overall fitness plan includes some form of cardio. Along with strength training it's the mainstay of most fitness programs. It's also the aspect of fitness most given to trends and fashions. In the 1980s we all got our cardio exercise from aerobics classes or Jane Fonda's workouts. In the early '90s, it was all about the Stairmaster and inline skating. Then came Tae Bo. Today, it's spin classes and "boot camps."

Lately, we've noticed a run of messaging against long cardio sessions and in favour of heavy weight training combined with high-intensity interval training (HIIT) instead. HIIT is quick bursts of very high effort, high intensity, followed by slightly longer (but by no means long) periods of rest. Workouts are shorter and, advocates claim, more efficient. HIIT is a response to the worry that cardio takes away all the muscle you gain from strength training. Some people even claim that cardio should be avoided because it "makes you fat." Sport does mean specialization—elite marathoners won't be world-class powerlifters. But if you're more of a generalist, with an interest in improving your overall fitness, cardio exercise isn't going away. Nor should it. If you want to draw up a well-rounded list of functional fitness skills, it has to include some sort of repeated movement that challenges your cardiovascular system.

So, what lurks behind the worry that "cardio makes you fat"? It used to be part of the common wisdom that if you were interested in losing weight you should do more (and more and *more*) cardio. It also used to be that "getting fit" meant losing weight. How could we forget? Of course, we challenge that equation—getting fit means a lot more than losing weight. But does steady cardio achieve that goal? Here's the thing: steady-state cardio at a relaxed pace for long periods of time won't produce the kind of fitness gains most people are looking for. Take running. Running long distances slowly and *only* running long distances slowly makes you good at exactly one thing. Yes, you guessed it: running long distances slowly.

Recent research on the benefits of HIIT is striking. High-intensity interval training—alternating between short bursts of anaerobic effort at close to your maximum heart rate and longer periods of recovery—has been shown to be effective at producing big gains in fitness with much less time spent training. For the time-strapped mid-life athlete, juggling the demands of family and work, HIIT is worth pursuing.

The most famous HIIT study was conducted at McMaster University in Hamilton, Ontario. Researchers found that cyclists doing one minute all-out sprints, with one minute recovery, ten times (that's just 20 minutes total) three times a week (just one hour a week) achieved the same training effect as they would riding ten hours at a moderate pace. That's dramatic: one hour a week instead of ten! But going all out is tough, even if only for a minute at a time. Not everyone can do that. So the researchers retested with intense but not all-out efforts. Even these less intense intervals yielded tremendous gains in fitness. They achieved a result that would take many more hours cycling at a lower speed and effort.

High-intensity exercise is a popular topic in exercise science and a hot trend among those who work out. It was crowned the top fitness trend for 2014, based on an annual worldwide survey conducted by the influential health and fitness organization the American College of Sports Medicine. It's tough, but you get results.

How can you make these findings work for you? Combining HIIT with more traditional long, slow approaches seems to offer the most benefits. The advantages of adding some intensity to your workouts are time efficiency and reducing the risk of injury from repetitive training. Remember that there is more to fitness than long sessions on the stationary bike—not that that doesn't have its upside (case in point: Tracy's summer spent reading *War and Peace*). No need to ditch the more endurance-oriented cardio entirely. Just mix it up with some big pushes.

When we cross-train, we mix things up by doing different activities. Just as HIIT combined with slower training sessions brings maximum benefit because it adds diversity, the variety of cross-training enables cardiovascular health to improve without taxing the same body parts and muscle groups over and over. For example, it's no secret that running can take its toll on the muscles and joints in our legs. But if a runner could reduce mileage and add some laps in the pool, that would work the heart and lungs while giving the legs a rest. This is why injury prevention is often cited as one of the key reasons to cross-train. Besides that, it's a great way to engage in "active recovery," which is a form of recovery from a previous workout that involves light activity of a different kind. And when we cross-train, we're less likely to get bored from the repetition and monotony of doing one thing over and over.

As for what to choose, you can get your cardio in all sorts of different ways, from trampoline jumping to cross-country skiing, from rowing to pole walking, from classes at the gym to hiking in the woods. During the FB50 Challenge we focused our attention on three main activities: biking, running, and swimming. And that's what the rest of this chapter is about. You? Do what you love, and mix it up.

Women Unite! Take Back the Bike! A Brief History of Women and Cycling

Women and bicycles have a long and fascinating history. Indeed, bicycling and feminism have been best friends if not forever, at least since the late 1800s, when bicycling provided the modern woman with independent transportation, playing a key role in the liberation of women. Advocates for women's cycling to this day quote Susan B. Anthony, who notoriously waxed poetic about women and bicycles, saying she thought the bicycle had "done more to emancipate women than anything else in the world."

How did the bicycle help with women's emancipation? With the bicycle came what was called "clothing reform." Imagine trying to ride in long skirts and petticoats. Safe and practical? Not so much. Wearing bloomers symbolized women's liberation from restrictive clothing and norms. It gave women the option of leaving the home in clothes that made movement practical. Naysayers opposed to women's newfound freedom harassed women cyclists because of their clothing. Women on bikes had few choices: some went so far as to dress as men to avoid being harassed while riding while also avoiding having to wear difficult clothes. That was the preferred strategy of women riding long distances.

So many women were riding bikes, shedding their restrictive clothing, and enjoying their new independence that an anti-bicycle backlash focused on women's liberation sprung up. "The New

Woman," as she was called, no longer knew her place (shocking!), and clergy and politicians taught the lesson that women risked their morals and their health by riding bikes.

Clergy preached about the moral corruption made possible by the bicycle as if the only thing standing between women and a life of sexual depravity, infidelity, and prostitution was reliable transport. Doctors worried that women might be biking for the purposes of sexual stimulation, that bicycling would lead to a corruption of the uterus, and, worse yet, that women would fall prey to the dreaded bicycle face (an actual medical ailment of the late 1800s associated with bicycle riding, caused by "excessive worry over maintaining balance while riding"). Many physicians proclaimed that women's bodies simply weren't suited to cycling. The bicycle was a sure path to sexual depravity and infertility. Also, poor weak women, so prone to exhaustion—how could biking possibly be a good choice for them?

Between the clothing, the independence, and the suitability of women's bodies for the strenuous nature of cycling, there was as much social anxiety about women on bicycles as the numbers of women willing to jump on their bikes and say, "Wheee!"

When It Comes to Bikes, Girls and Women Still Don't Own Half the Road

That was then. What about today? Bikes still stand for women's freedom. Some places still deter women from riding bikes. The 2012 Saudi Arabian film *Wadjda* tells the story of a determined young girl who takes part in a Qur'an recitation contest in order to win enough money to purchase a green bike so she can beat her friend Abdullah in a race. Wadjda goes after the bike even though the law prohibits unchaperoned women from riding bikes in public. The film caused controversy in Saudi Arabia over worries that it would incite change, for instance, in the way women dress, like the rational dress movement had in England and North America. In 2013 Saudi Arabia dropped the ban on women riding bikes. Saudi Arabian women are now permitted to ride in parks and "recreational areas"—as long as they wear full body coverings and are accompanied by a male relative.

Bikes have the potential to change the lives of girls when it comes to education, too. In "Cycling to School: Increasing Secondary School Enrollment for Girls in India," Karthik Muralidharan and Nishith Prakash show how bikes can keep girls in school. In rural India about half of all girls drop out midway through their education. School is free, but transportation isn't. As the authors explain, if you give a bike to a girl who would otherwise have to leave school, she gets to stay in school. NGOs like Give a Girl a Bike work to make this happen in rural India.

But what about in the West? Do we have bike equality and equality through the bike? That's debatable. Studies show that cycling is still a man's sport in which women struggle for equal status. That's true both in racing and in everyday cycling or bike commuting.

Consider the kilo. In track cycling, the 1,000-metre time trial ("the kilo" for short) is considered the toughest event. "Probably the most painful of track disciplines," one guide to track racing describes it. It's widely believed by cyclists to be the hardest distance—a good time for an elite racer is just over one minute. At the UCI Track Cycling World Championships, only senior men race the kilo. Junior men and women race 500 metres and not the kilo. A woman might race the kilo at the club level, but it makes no sense for women to train for this distance as there are no licensed racing events that include the option for women. The time trial was removed from the Olympics program after 2004, in both its 500 metre and kilo version, but these distances remain for track cycling at national and other international levels.

Then there's the Tour. The toughest road bike race in the world is thought to be the Tour de France, which isn't labelled as a *men's* cycling event but, in fact, is. Women's cycling seems not to have the support of the bike-racing community or fans. There is a tour labelled as the "Women's Tour," but while men's bike racing seems to be enjoying an upsurge in popularity, the tour formerly known as the Tour Cycliste Féminin, or simply Tour Féminin, hasn't been held since 2008.

You might think this is just a problem at the professional level that doesn't need to bother amateurs. But what's telling about how entrenched the attitudes to women on bikes are is that the sexism in cycling goes all the way down, from pro events to amateur cycling competitions. In amateur events in cycling distances often vary drastically between men's and women's. So too does the prize money. A recent Atlanta 100K race dramatically showcases both of these inequalities. The women's event is a 10-kilometre race with a $2,000 payout. The men's race is 100 kilometres and pays $10,000.

Discomfort about women on bikes goes past racing at all levels. Even everyday cyclists and bike commuters aren't removed from it when it comes to the topic of suitable clothing. Recent opposition to bike lanes in Brooklyn, New York, was due to the fact that the bike lanes would have gone through orthodox Jewish neighbourhoods. Hasidic leaders complained that with women biking around in shorts, they would have trouble obeying their religious law forbidding them from staring at members of the opposite sex.

So while it might look as if the attitudes to women's cycling which we associate with the 1800s are long past, in fact they're still around, both in competitive cycling and everyday commuting and casual riding.

"If you want to know if an urban environment supports cycling, you can forget about all the detailed 'bikeability indexes'—just measure the proportion of cyclists who are female," says Australian researcher Jan Garrard.[1] In the U.S. in 2009, men made the twice the number of cycling trips as women. In Europe, meanwhile, urban biking had become a way of life, about as many women rode as men. In the Netherlands, where 27% of trips were made by bike, it was over half. There, 55% of riders were women.

Garrard was also one of three women professors—of urban planning, health, and environmental science—who contributed a chapter together to a volume on urban cycling.[2] Women, they say, are an "indicator species" for bike-friendly cities. In cities and countries where a high percentage of bike trips are by women, rates of cycling are high and cycling conditions are safe, convenient, and comfortable. Where relatively few women cycle, rates of cycling are low and cycling conditions are unsafe, inconvenient, uncomfortable, and sometimes impossible.

Discomfort about seeing women on bicycles continues to this day. Bike racing is an incredibly male-dominated sport. Yet the bicycle continues to play a role in women's liberation around the globe, whether it's helping girls get to school in India or providing independent travel for women in Saudi Arabia, where bike riding is allowed but driving a car is currently not. (Saudi Arabia's King Salman issued a royal decree in September 2017 that will allow women to drive beginning June 24, 2018.) Bike riding is also an important positive change we can make to help the environment and help make our cities more livable, and girls and women have a crucial role to play.

It's as Easy as Riding a Bike: Getting Fit on Two Wheels

Chances are you learned to ride a bike as a child. Most of us know how to ride a bike. But why start again as an adult? Cycling is an excellent way to increase your cardiovascular fitness, whether you ride as part of everyday exercise (commuting to work, running errands), as a specific training regimen (aiming to increase speed or distance, or both), or as a social activity involving long rides in the countryside to look at the scenery and drink coffee in new locations.

While running, swimming, rowing, and riding are all good cardio-enhancing activities, there are some advantages specific to riding a bike. It's easier on your joints than running, and unlike running, it's not primarily a weight-bearing exercise (hills are the one exception). If you're starting out on your fitness journey as a larger person, biking can be the way to go. Cycling also builds muscle strength and improves your balance and coordination.[3]

For those of us who love cycling, riding a bike is also a great way to perk up our mood. Cycling certainly makes Sam smile, and lots of studies show the mental health benefits of riding a bike.[4]

See How She Runs: How Women Have Changed the Face of Running

Outside of the local running shop, runners lean up against the bike rack to stretch out their calves or pull their foot up behind them to loosen up their quads. Winter or summer, rain or shine, in the daylight or the dark of night they show up, some in fancy tights, others in baggy shorts. Running is the most visible and popular fitness activity in our culture these days. More people are running marathons than ever before and the average finishing time is increasing along with the participation rate. Training with a race in mind, from a 5K to a marathon or beyond, whether you're an elite runner or a first-timer, is a great way to commit to a consistent schedule. Besides the simplicity of it, running is fantastic and efficient cardio and great for reducing stress.

But the story of women's running is another story of exclusion. Organized races were for men. People thought women's constitutions were too delicate for strenuous activity. Yadda, yadda, yadda. These biases show up in the way that women-specific sports developed. Netball, for example, is a "female-friendly" version of basketball, and one of the main changes is that in netball you don't move with the ball—you throw it to a teammate. The upshot: less running. In England, Australia, and New Zealand, netball remains a popular sport for women instead of basketball. Does basketball really have too much running for women to handle? We wouldn't want to put such frail creatures at risk now, would we? Remember when they used to keep menstruating girls on the sidelines in gym? All that running around could jeopardize their reproductive health. Their uteruses might fall out from the impact. Strenuous exertion could draw the blood away from the female reproductive organs, rendering them useless. That's really what people thought ... and not so long ago, either. We're going to go out on a limb here and say: don't worry about it.

Marathons are now everywoman events, but that's a recent shift. The first American woman to officially finish a marathon was Arlene Pieper, in 1959 in Manitou Springs, Colorado. On the 50th anniversary of her milestone race, Pieper, by then 83, said in an interview, "Back then, women weren't allowed to do much. I wanted to run the Boston Marathon, but they wouldn't let me. We were just supposed to stay home, bake cookies, and have babies."

Kathrine Switzer broke into the prestigious Boston Marathon officially (with a number) in 1967. She trained for the event after her coach told her the marathon distance was too far for "fragile women." But it's not as if the race organizers would have let her in if they'd *known* she wasn't a man. Switzer entered using only her initials. Race organizers tried to throw her off the course for racing in "flagrant violation of the rules." Many of us know Switzer's story and have seen the iconic image of a race official attempting to eject her. It took another 15 years, until 1984, for the women's marathon to become part of the summer Olympics.

Today, women fuel the popularity of running. In the United States each year the number of people running hits a new high, and women make up the majority of the new runners. If running endangers the uterus, most of us didn't get the memo. In 2013 a record-setting 19 million people finished U.S. running events, according to Running USA—that's an increase of 300% since 1990, with women making up nearly 60% of those running. If you'd rather stick with the women, women-only races and women-only running clinics abound.

Why might running be a good choice for you? It lures people in because of the low cost and the simplicity of it. All you need is a pair of running shoes (sort of—we confess that this may be an exaggeration, but you can get away with way less gear than other activities demand). And it's easy to fit running into a busy schedule. Squeeze in that run before the rest of the family wakes up. Step out the door for a half an hour before your morning shower. Do some hill repeats after work. Maybe, like Tracy, you love the social side of running. It's really easy to chat while you run, at least on those slow, long Sunday-morning runs with friends. The run-and-talk outing is like an amped-up version of meeting the crew for a latte. Lots of running groups go out for coffee after the run. Tracy and her running peeps do a post-run breakfast every so often. And you can run for all manner of charitable causes—no need to have competition as your motive. How about running for the cure for breast cancer, for diabetes, or for retina research?

Some commentators attribute some of the changes in running culture to the rise in the numbers of women taking part. What sorts of changes? First, the rise of the "participation" event as opposed to the "competitive" event. Get doused with neon powder in a colour run. Do a down and dirty obstacle course on a mud run. Or take in a different kind of nightlife at a night-run event with bright lights and fluorescent body paint. Sam did an adventure race a few years ago in which the obstacles that involved cool water on a hot day were so welcome and fun that people were lining up to do them again. Finishing times didn't rank as the highest priority for that group. If you have a penchant for the theatrical, you can embark on a running adventure where you're fleeing zombies or prison guards. Or you can even get risqué with an X-rated adult race (what happens at the X-rated race, stays at the X-rated race).

Aside from the X-rated race, themed races often make an explicit appeal to involve family members. Some of the zombie races allow you to bring children along and sign them in as zombies—older children can be the speedy chasing zombies and younger children can be painted up as "stumbler" zombies. This lighthearted attitude toward running now even permeates more serious events. In recent years, it's rare to take part in any event without seeing someone running in a funny hat or a tutu.

The mass participation events have fuelled a mix of fitness and tourism where people, many of them women with a group of friends, travel to a fun destination to run a race. At Disney you can sign up for the Goofy Challenge, where you run a half marathon on Saturday and a full marathon on Sunday, or the Dopey

Challenge, where on consecutive days you run a 5K, 10K, half marathon, and full marathon, all through the park. If you're into ultras—distances beyond the 42-kilometre marathon—you can do 50K at Burning Man in the Nevada desert at the end of August. And of course urban races, where you get to run through the streets of cities like Chicago, New York, or San Francisco, are so popular they sell out each year.

Even events without a fun feature—no mud, no zombies, no spray-on colour—have gone wild with themes and swag bags. The Niagara Women's Half Marathon boasts wine from the region as part of the loot. The 2015 Nike 15K in Toronto subbed in tasteful necklaces that competitors might actually wear in lieu of medals that just hang on a hook on the back of the closet door, never to be donned again.

Repeat after us: The success of women in running isn't just about participation. At the level of ultra running, women are taking the lead—winning. Against male competitors, too. At the marathon level, the very best women would come 20th if ranked against the men, but at races over 160 kilometres, the overall winners are often women. Why? There's speculation about women's success in ultra events. Part of the story is that women are physically smaller and the longer the race, the more size matters. The causal story also seems to involve our higher body fat percentage and the ability of our bodies to use fat as fuel when we run. Again, the longer the distance, the more that matters.

So it's a mistake to tell the story of women and running as primarily a story of mass participation. For sure, it's true that more women are running than ever before and that the numbers of everyman and everywoman athletes have changed the culture of running. But if you just look at that piece you miss some of the tremendous gains that women runners are making. Other barriers are falling down too. Women are setting new records at older ages and at longer distances.

The women masters runners are an amazing part of the story, setting new records for speed at a given age each year. Olga

Kotelko, a retired schoolteacher, *started* running at age 77. In her mid-90s she was still setting records on the track. Sister Madonna Buder, the Iron Nun, at 85 holds the record for being the oldest person to complete an Iron distance triathlon. Buder started competing in her late 40s and has finished more than 325 triathlons of various distances. She is also an excellent model for fitting exercise into one's life. She runs or bikes to church and to the prison where she reads scripture to inmates.

In *Older Faster Stronger: What Women Runners Can Teach Us All about Living, Younger Longer,* Margaret Webb asks whether there is an evolutionary reason that women can continue to run, train, and maintain endurance in our advanced years. She notes that large numbers of women, like Kotelko and Buder, are taking up running in later life.

Whether it's the Badwater 100 or your neighbourhood 5K coffee run, more women are out there running longer and running older than ever before. We can both see this in our own lives. Tracy has developed some super close friendships through running, all with women who started running in their 40s and 50s. Some are faster, some are slower, but all of us are out there pounding the pavement alone and in groups several times a week.

Splish Splash: Women Take to the Water

Swimming is another repetitive, easy-access activity that has tons of potential as a cardio workout, a stress release, and an endurance sport. As a no-impact activity, it's gentler on the bones and joints than running. Time in the pool really counts. In a recent step challenge Tracy did at work, she got to cash in every 1,000 metres in the pool for 4,750 steps. That meant that whenever she went for an early-morning swim, she easily clocked over 10,000 by 8 a.m.

Swimming has its challenges if you're learning later in life. You have to get your stroke right, and equally important, you need to learn a whole new breathing pattern that coordinates with your stroke. That's why swimming does wonders for cardiovascular fitness. An efficient freestyle swimmer will exhale completely under water and inhale deeply on every third stroke (thus alternating sides, which makes more "gears" available and helps keep you swimming in a straighter line because you're not favouring one side). This breathing rhythm helps the lungs and heart to move oxygen efficiently and to make the heart stronger.

Swimming engages the whole body, working all major muscle groups. It increases flexibility and muscular endurance at the same time. It engages the core, which in turn strengthens the hips, lower back, and abdominal muscles.

With no impact, it's the perfect recovery activity for endurance runners. After Tracy ran her first marathon (post FB50 Challenge), her triathlon coach recommended that she swim during the week following to "kick out" her legs. Because swimming takes the load off the legs and highlights the upper body more than running or cycling, it's a good choice for cross-training. If you're not yet a swimmer, don't let the steep learning curve put you off. It's worth it.

Like cycling and running, there's an odd history of women and the water. How many of us have sat on the sidelines while the rest of the kids swam? It was a myth, propagated by high school teachers and camp counsellors everywhere back in the '70s, that menstruating women shouldn't swim. Maybe it was more about the awkwardness of trying to fix an adhesive pad onto a swimsuit back in the day, when the pads were an inch thick and unlikely to stay stuck once they got wet. Or maybe it was a concern about recommending tampons to kids who (everyone hoped) were virgins. Some sources even talk about the fear that leaking menstrual blood might lure sharks, making women and girls on their periods more susceptible to attack (which doesn't help explain anything about not swimming in lakes or swimming pools, but never mind). Whatever the reasons, this familiar myth that swimming and periods don't mix well took hold in the popular imagination. And somehow it got translated into the idea that menstruating girls and women ought to stay out of the pool.

That story has not been totally laid to rest. Today, if you do a web search for "swimming" and "menstruation," you'll land on a plethora of pages dedicated to debunking the myth and making recommendations about how to swim with your period. Check out the WikiHow "How to Swim When You Are on Your Period." The short answer: wear a tampon.

Another potential downside that keeps women away from swimming is that it requires perhaps the most minimalist of all workout wear: the swimsuit. Tight, revealing clothing has proven to be a deterrent for women wishing to engage in physical activities. For some sports there may be options, but swimming allows few alternatives. Every spring, we are inundated with messages about how to get our "beach body" or our "bikini body." And every spring, we see counter-messages like "Your beach body is the body you take to the beach." If you can take that attitude with you to the pool, then despite the fact that swimming means donning a body-hugging suit, you have a year-round activity that has all sorts of other benefits.

It used to be that women's swimwear options were limited in a different way. If you're on social media, you may have seen the striking 1922 photo, colourised by Patty Allison, of the swimsuit police taking a tape measure to the space between the top of a woman's knee and the bottom of the skirt of her swimsuit. A suit more than six inches above knee was a no-go. This paranoia about swimsuits and "indecent exposure" required women in the early twentieth century to wear a long, one-piece bathing suit and, in some jurisdictions, even stockings to cover their bare legs.

So while some of us might feel hesitant about the body-hugging quality of the modern swimsuit, the alternative of having modesty forced upon us would be more unwelcome. Wearing a swimsuit unselfconsciously makes a statement about body comfort, sport-appropriate clothing, and a woman's right to wear functional and suitable attire that allows her to engage safely and comfortably in her chosen sports.

Let's say you decide to give swimming a try. How do you get started? Most urban areas have local pools with regular schedules of lane swimming and masters groups you can train with. It's not as easy to pick up as running if you didn't learn to swim as a child. But it's not impossible to find adult swim lessons, coaches who are willing to work with you one-on-one to improve your stroke, and clinics to teach new methods of achieving efficiency in the water. One such technique is total immersion swimming, a favourite of triathletes for its emphasis on reducing drag, streamlining to glide through the water farther and faster with less effort, and conserving energy.

These days, a lot of people have a renewed interest in swimming because it's one of three disciplines in the most popular multisport event: triathlon. Triathlon has cross-training built right into it.

For the Woman Who Wants More: Triathlon

You've seen lots about triathlon in earlier chapters and in Tracy's personal story. You may recall how she surprised herself in year one of our FB50 Challenge by falling in love with triathlon, when she had gone in thinking her foray into that world was just a one-off to give her something to blog about. What's great about triathlon training is that it requires cross-training, so if you go for triathlon you're automatically going to get variety. You'll swim, bike, and run your way to cardio fitness no matter which distance lures you in.

If you're thinking about trying triathlon, look for smaller races in your area that offer "give-it-a-tri" or "try-a-tri" events. These cater to newbies and that makes them more fun, less intense, than any other distance. At all other distances, you'll find a range of competitors, from elites who tear up the course to everyday athletes who take at least twice as long to finish.

Here's something else about cardio and the importance of cross-training in case you're wondering why we're so gung ho about mixing things up. In a word: injury. If you cross-train, you are less likely to have to sit out with an injury. Sam started in her 40s as a runner and only when she took up triathlon did she realize she was actually a much faster cyclist. When running injuries eventually took her out of triathlon, she kept right on cycling. When you cross-train, you've always got other activities as backup. Not just that, though. Variety gives your body a break from working the same muscles in the same way over and over and over again. Some people think you only have so many kilometres of running available to you in a lifetime. If you spread those kilometres out over many years by sprinkling them in with other activities, you might be able to run for a lot longer.

Take it away...
Women have long been encouraged to do lengthy sessions of steady-state cardio, often on machines at the gym. Instead, think about cross-training—choosing a variety of activities that get the heart rate up—as a way of mixing up the routine and discovering new activities that spark joy.

Try this...
Use this time of life—whatever time of life you're in—to add some cross-training to your repertoire. If you're a runner, try adding some time on the bike. If you're a swimmer already, how about learning to run? Or if you've ever felt curious about triathlon, find a local club. There are lots and they welcome newbies.

TWELVE

The FB50 Challenge

One Year to 18 Months—
Tracy's and Sam's Stories

Tracy's Story: Getting Serious about Triathlon Training

A year into the challenge, my goal took shape as I caught a serious case of triathlon fever. I ventured out beyond the safety of the all-women's event in Kincardine to do the shortest distance on offer at the Lakeside triathlon weekend that September. From there, the momentum of triathlon training gathered force. Over the next six months I got serious about swimming, biking, and running as I set a new target for my FB50 Challenge: to complete at least one Olympic distance triathlon before my 50th birthday.

September and October 2013: Giving-It-a-Tri, Resetting My FB50 Goal, and Taking the Plunge

Kincardine gave me the multisport bug, but Lakeside was the real thing. Even though I had only signed up for the "Give-it-a-Tri," the triathlon at Lakeside is a huge, serious event, with a bunch of different distances of triathlon and duathlon over the weekend. It's not women-only, either. Lakeside, Ontario, is close to home with a small and shallow lake at no risk of being too cold to pass official triathlon rules for minimum water temperatures. You know that feeling where you can't quite tell the difference between excitement and fear? That's what I had in the two weeks leading up to Lakeside.

The Lakeside Give-It-a-Tri is a super-short course: 375 metres in the water, 10K on the bike, and a 2.5K run. The whole point of it is to give newbies the experience of multisport. I knew I'd finish, but it felt like a serious event, not the fun times of Kincardine. My niece and fellow tri-er Jolene picked me up early on a cold, wet morning. The weather had broken a bit by the time we got to Lakeside. There was lots of nervous laughter between the two of us as we wheeled our bikes from the car to the transition area. Everyone entering the area with a bike had to get a wristband with a matching marker to go around the bike seat post. Someone would check these at the end, when we packed up to go home. Apparently, earlier that summer a bike had been stolen at an event in Ottawa. To my surprise, the person giving out the bands was Gabbi Whitlock, who I knew from work. Gabbi worked at the university but also founded and ran a local triathlon club, Balance Point Triathlon, where she did (and does) group and one-on-one coaching. I felt relieved and embarrassed at the same time: relieved because it's great to see a friendly face at these things, embarrassed because I didn't know what I was doing and now someone I actually knew would see me in all of my novice, untrained, know-nothing glory. I didn't even expect to be able to run 2.5K without stopping.

I used a borrowed wetsuit for the swim, breaking one of the first rules of wetsuits: never try one on for the first time on race day. At least I was smart enough to keep the flat pedals on for the race rather than try to speed-learn how to ride with clipless pedals. Learning to ride with clipless pedals a few weeks later turned out to be a painful experience, so that was a good decision.

If you're going to try triathlon for the first time, definitely do a "try-a-tri" type of event. That way you won't feel nearly as foolish about asking basic questions, like "How do I rack my bike?" Jolene and I set ourselves up in the transition area and then went to the beach to pull on our wetsuits and listen to the pre-race meeting to get an overview of the course. I followed a wetsuit tip I'd read: put plastic bags over your feet and then your hands to make it easier to pull on the suit. It worked like a dream. Suit slid on and I was ready to go! Unfortunately, a few of us had a mix-up with our timing chips and didn't have a chance for a practice swim—not recommended. A few strokes before the race starts make all the difference.

There's a buzz in the air before any event, and the Lakeside Give-It-a-Tri was no different. As we gathered on the beach awaiting our starts, with Jolene in the wave before me because she's quite a bit younger, the tension rose. I heard lots of apprehensive titters around me. As start time approached, Jolene and I hugged and wished each other well.

Next thing you know, she was off. And not long after that, I was heading into the water surrounded by about 50 other people in the "40 and over" wave, trying to carve out a spot for myself while keeping to the right of the big neon green floating cones that marked the course. I'd felt confident about the swim before stepping into the lake because even though I hadn't trained much (okay, at all) for speed, swimming was my most comfortable event. The advice about not letting race day be the first time you swim in a wetsuit has merit, though. The suit constricted my range of motion, and wetsuits give you a kind of buoyancy that's good but that takes some getting used to. On top of that, I struggled to find my rhythm and catch my breath, despite the fact that I'm usually a really rhythmic swimmer who has no difficulty with the breathing part. And through the murky water (ew!) I could see weeds (double ew!).

My aversion to weeds kicked me into high gear as I rounded the second cone to head toward shore. I came out further ahead than

I'd expected. As suggested, I peeled the wetsuit down to my waist as I headed to the transition area for my first triathlon T1. You know how your heart just pounds when you're doing something a little bit daring? That's how I felt as I stepped out of the wetsuit and pulled socks over wet feet, slipped into my shoes, donned my bike helmet, and snapped on the strap (you're not allowed even to touch your bicycle until you've done that). I ran to the mount line.

Underway on the bike, I sped along, passing some people and being passed by others. I'd had my new bike in my possession for about 24 hours (also not recommended!) and had to learn quickly which gears did what. I wouldn't call it the most efficient ride of my life, but oh well—10K later, I pulled the brakes at the dismount line and ran with my bike back to the transition area for T2. It's a faster transition, especially if you don't need to change your shoes. I just racked the bike, dumped the helmet and started running.

I didn't feel like it at all. My legs felt as if they were filled with lead and resisted moving the way they're supposed to move. That's normal for the transition from biking to running. I forced myself out of the transition area to run-walk what was possibly the slowest 2.5K of my life. And when I made it across the finish line? I felt giddy with the experience of having completed an actual, bona fide triathlon, even if a teeny-tiny triathlon, and even if I came in 8th out of 10 in my age group, 133 out of 155 overall. Not stellar, not pretty, but I did it. Jolene finished ahead of me but decided that was it for her and triathlon. But me? I was already formulating a plan.

Remember Gabbi, the familiar face I saw when I entered the transition area at Lakeside to set up for the race? She's an amazing coach with all sorts of triathlon experience herself. Not long after Lakeside, as I ruminated about my triathlon goals, I set up a meeting with Gabbi to talk about possibilities. She said that she thought I could realistically set an Olympic distance triathlon as a goal. The Olympic distance is significantly longer than anything I'd done so far, even in the individual components. It's a 1,500-metre swim, a 40-kilometre bike ride, and a 10K run. The swim I knew I could handle, but I'd never ridden 40K or run 10K. Gabbi said, "With training, no problem."

Training—that was a new concept to me. So far, I'd been dabbling. Not so long before Lakeside I had considered triathlon just a one-time thing to do on a lark. But now, just a month into the second year of our FB50 Challenge, I set a new goal: to swim farther than I'd ever swum, bike farther than I'd ever biked, and run farther than I'd ever run.

Gabbi told me, "The first thing you need to do is sign up for my triathlon swim group at the Y." On a Tuesday morning at the end of September I showed up on the pool deck at 6 a.m. for my first group swimming endeavour since I'd taken lessons as a child. The group met twice a week, but I only committed to once because at that point I had a weekly 6:30 a.m. yoga class competing for my attention. In the first days of my triathlon training, I still thought I could do all that—run three times a week, *and* keep up the pace with yoga and weight training.

And then there was the bike. If you keep your flat pedals on your road bike, you kill the bike's full potential. Clipless pedals (which is a confusing name because you have to clip into them with special cleated shoes) give a better power transfer. It makes sense when you think about it. With flat pedals, you're only getting power to the bike when you push down. But when your feet are attached to the pedal, as with clipless, you can push on the downside of the rotation and pull up on the upside of the rotation. The double benefit of this system is that you get more continuous power to the bike and at the same time you engage different muscles, as the core and hip flexors kick in for the upstroke. So it's more efficient and you save some of the running muscles for the run.

When you're clipped into your pedals, it's like being snapped into the bindings on skis or a snowboard. That direct connection gives great control and power transfer. But most of us who haven't done that before find it kind of terrifying to be locked in like that. And I was no different. It's one thing to practise clipping in and out in the store, when your bike is securely on a trainer and can't fall over. But that's just the beginning.

Let's just say I had a painful initiation into that kind of riding. On my first try, I ventured out to the laneway behind my house *alone,* thinking, *How hard can this be?* Turns out it can be plenty hard. Hard like the asphalt in the laneway. Hard like, ouch, if I fall on that elbow one more time I'm going to curl up right here, in the laneway, beside my bike and cry. Hard like, I think I'm going to faint before I can drag myself and my bike back to the shed.

I clipped the one foot in, as directed. But then I was confused about what to do next. As my right foot flailed unclipped in the air, desperately trying to make contact with the pedal, I forgot some simple physics: the bike needs forward motion to stay upright. Just a couple of days before I had cavalierly said to Sam that I just didn't understand how someone could fall the opposite way, away from the unclipped foot to the clipped foot side, when they had one foot free. Why wouldn't you just put the unclipped foot down?

Well, within mere minutes of "trying this at home," I understood. With my right foot flailing around, I ever so slowly started to fall to the left. Helpless to stop myself, I landed on my elbow. Then I kind of lay there for a few seconds because my bottom foot was, of course, still clipped in. I lifted the bike enough to unclip, picked myself and the bike up, and went to the shed to hold onto the wall and practise clipping in and out again.

But I was stationary. That's easy. Back to the laneway (or rather the driveway—this time I didn't feel ready to venture off the property). I managed to get going, I even stopped successfully. But then when I tried again, same thing as before. Boom. That's when I saw stars and felt like I was going to faint. My one recommendation: ask for help. I did. That's when Sam came to the rescue.

Sam met me in the park the next morning. I had on my full-armour motorcycle jacket from when I used to ride my Yamaha 650. Sam vetoed my suggestion to practise on the grass—too uneven and you have to clip in at speed.

She broke it down the way she had when she taught kids at her bike club in Australia. Step one: Learn to coast with one foot clipped in and to put down the dominant foot when you stop (that's key if you don't want to topple over, helplessly, the wrong way like I did). Step two: Learn how to pedal with one foot. This keeps things leisurely. No rush about clipping in the second foot if you can pedal through an intersection with just the one foot clipped in. Take your time. Step three: Clip the second foot in and out at speed. It's really not so hard once you've got the coasting and the one-footed pedalling figured out. Clipping in is a matter of lining up your shoe cleat with the pedal and snapping it in. Clipping out requires a little twist of the heel. With the right instructions from Sam, I had it figured out in less than half an hour, just in time for fall riding season.

On my first long bike ride that fall, Sam and another very experienced bike friend of ours, Jacquie, tried to teach me how to draft. Drafting is when you ride close to the rear wheel of the rider in front. The front rider blocks the wind, creating less resistance for the rider behind. According to statistics, drafting can reduce wind resistance by as much as 27%. Riding with a group can require up to 40% less energy expenditure than riding alone. But every time I approached one of their rear wheels, I went into a quiet panic. Jacquie assured me that nothing bad would happen to the front rider if I hit their rear wheel. I was more worried about what would happen to *me,* the back rider. For drafting, I would need practice.

Sam flattered me with her generous assumptions about what I was capable of on the bike. That first day, she dragged me out (that's how it felt) for a 50-kilometre ride when the farthest I'd ever ridden before that was the 12K in Kincardine. I had work to do if I was going to gain speed and endurance. The thing with being the slowest person in the group is that, if you're like me, you worry that you're holding everyone up. Sam assured me that someone is always the slowest in the group and that most groups are fine with that. You just change your pace and be willing to wait. But seasoned cyclists are speedy, especially at the end of a long season of riding, so I felt self-conscious at just how slow I was. There wasn't a lot I could do about it (other than master drafting, which still to this day I have not). So I exhausted myself trying to ride as fast I could, and they still waited for me at the top of every hill and at each intersection.

The first sign that I may not take to the bike in the way I'd hoped: I liked the post-ride coffee and cake much more than the ride itself. I just wish we'd stopped closer to home, because I had a lot of trouble getting back on my bike to ride another 10 kilometres after that.

If riding a road bike is new to you, find a group of friends, at least some with proper group riding experience (etiquette and technique are key to riding with a group so you want people who can pass the conventions on to you), build up to longer distances gradually (no matter what your friends think you might be able to do), and make sure there's some social time around food built into it somewhere along the way.

November and December 2013: Swimming, Biking, and Ramping Up the Running

I'd had high hopes for the bike, but during those early days of more serious triathlon training, it was the swim sessions that lit the fire in me. Even though swimming with a group was all new to me, within no time at all I could see the many benefits of this approach to my training. For one thing, signing up for stuff makes me commit. If you're like me, you don't just throw away your money. If I'm paying, I'm much more likely to go. And I loved that it was early enough in the morning that I could get in my workout, stretch in the steam room, shower, and still be home in time to have breakfast with Renald at 8 a.m. Swimming with a group gives you a sense of relative speed. We did time trials and gauged our progress. And I got a grasp on where I stood in relation to others. We had four lanes of the pool, and I was in the second. That means there were two lanes of faster swimmers, and one lane of slower. I was among the faster swimmers in my lane, and for a while, I regularly took the lead. And that's another benefit: being ahead of others in a lane makes you swim faster and push harder. As a swimmer, the only thing worse than being stuck behind someone swimming too slowly is feeling the person behind you touching your feet with their hands. Then *you're* the tortoise holding up the traffic!

Another bonus: It's really fun to swim with other people and meet others who care about swimming. I'd thought of swimming as a solitary activity, but after just a few weeks, I really started to feel a sense of camaraderie with my lane mates—so much so that now, after a few years of swimming with more or less the same group, we feel a bit sad when one of us "graduates" to the faster lane. It's like saying goodbye to a friend who is moving on to better things... bittersweet.

If all that good stuff's not enough, there's real inspiration in churning up the pool regularly with other triathletes. They get a kick out of sharing their experiences and talking about their plans for the season. I got to do my laps and drills with people training for everything from sprint distance to full distance and in between. Contagious focus like that creates a sense of wild possibility. Try it and see. Amid the early-morning chatter with lane mates—ordinary folks who had their own big plans and whose automatic response to anyone's ambitions, no matter how grand, was always "Way to go!" and "That's awesome!"—my ephemeral goal of doing the Olympic distance event as the pinnacle of my FB50 Challenge got real.

I approached the bike with some optimism even though owning a road bike, never mind riding with clipless pedals, had been on my "never" list until a week before Lakeside. If I could focus on the specific skills needed to get the most out of a road bike, maybe, just maybe, my phobia about the road would take care of itself. When I learned to ride with the clipless pedals, I thought I was all set. All I needed to do was get the mileage, as they say—spend time on the bike, on the road, logging some time and distance.

London, Ontario, is considered to have mostly flat cycling terrain with lots of rural roads, though by November, the wind really kicks in around our little city. I committed to giving the bike an honest try. The season ender for me happened one Sunday when I once again forced myself to go out with Sam and her friends. I'd been seriously hoping for a rain-out so I could just stay inside. Those November winds howled, gusting to 60 kilometres per hour, and the high for the day was only 6°C. I had no booties to keep my feet warm, so I taped up the air vents in my shoes with duct tape in the hopes my toes would not freeze.

They decided on the "Belmont short loop." If someone had told me in advance that "short" meant 50K, half of it into the wind, I would have bailed. But they didn't say that. I suffered through the worst bike ride of my life (ever). It included about half an hour of blissful tailwind, but the rest was pure suffering. I cursed the people I was riding with, as if they had planned this disastrous day. From cramped quads to toppling over on a hill, from a head-wind against which I felt I could hardly move to a harrowing ride through an industrial park where I was told to anticipate being chased by dogs (mercifully, that didn't happen), every brutal minute of that ride is forever etched into my memory.

Sam consoled me by pointing out that no one enjoyed the ride that day. Conditions were indeed awful, not just according to my own distorted standards. So it would be totally unfair for me to draw any conclusions about cycling based on that day. Less than a week later, however, it snowed. That marked the end of bike season for me.

I had too little time in the saddle to judge where I would end up with the bike. Despite some difficult outings, I felt solid on my bike and by the end of outdoor riding season the pedals posed no problem for me. Sam reported that I looked confident and skilled as a rider. That made sense to me—I had some transferable skills from my years of riding my motorcycle, both safety skills and road-handling skills, that served me well. Still, you can only do so much. Most cyclists and triathletes switch to indoor training when winter sets in, and in subsequent years I've done that too. But that year I just hung up the bike on its hook in the shed and turned my attention to running.

My group swimming experience had taught me the value of having set training commitments and training with others, so I signed up for a 10K training group through the Running Room, a store that specializes in running apparel and organizes running groups and events. We met as a closed group on Thursday evenings, and before our run someone would come in to talk to us about something to do with running—gear, shoes, nutrition, injury prevention. On Wednesdays and Sundays we joined the Running Room's regular run club. It's a great community of people of different levels of experience with an interest in running at all distances. Sunday is always the long run. What counts as "long" depends very much on which group you're training with. For the 10K people, we started off with 6K on the Sunday and worked our way all the way up to 13K, on the theory that you should train to exceed, not just meet, the distance of the event you're training for. This may be true of all distances up to the half marathon. It's less popular among the marathon-training crowd because 42 kilometres takes its toll on the body, so you probably don't want to do it more times than necessary.

The 10K group kept me going through the winter months. By the time the snow came in early December, there was many a Wednesday, Thursday, or Sunday where I would not have stepped foot out the door if I hadn't signed up for the group. I'd say one of my best qualities, boring though it may be, is my level of commitment once I've signed up for something. It's a rare day that I will skip out on a commitment. And even though we were just training for 10K, when there were marathon and half marathon folks doing much longer distances, I enjoyed the "we're all in this together" feeling on the snowy, windy nights of plowing through uncleared sidewalks. It makes you feel pretty hardcore.

January and February 2014: Nutrition and Race Sign-Ups

By January, I had my training routine humming along but I'd paid little attention to what I was eating. I'd been eating intuitively for a full year in the hopes of ridding myself once and for all of my chronic obsession with food and body weight. The year had done me a lot of good. It freed me up to focus on my physical training with nothing but performance in mind. No longer did I think of physical activity as a means to the one ultimate end of getting thinner. And I'd stopped weighing myself, which meant that I no longer let the number on the scale dictate how I felt. This was all good, a newfound freedom.

But at the same time, fact: nutrition is a component of good training. I'd learned in the running clinic, for example, about eating appropriately to fuel your runs in a way that doesn't load you down. I knew too that you can't do an Olympic distance event, where you would be out there for two to three hours, without eating something along the way. Sam had done an online nutrition coaching program the year before. She had mixed feelings about it because it paid a lot of attention to body weight. But its main virtue was a focus on healthy habits—not strict rules but regular behaviours that, when practised the majority of the time, would result in an overall healthy lifestyle. I'm wary of anything that promotes dieting as a "way of life," but a habits-based program seemed reasonable. I signed up for the year thinking I could benefit from that approach.

The program wasn't only about nutrition. It included a workout schedule each week, with three weight-training sessions, some interval training, active recovery, and a rest day. I had to tweak it a bit. They suggested Sunday as a rest day, but that was when my 10K group did its long run. With my swimming, running, and yoga, I cut the weight training down from three sessions a week to two. Otherwise, it would have been more than my schedule could bear. By then, I'd dropped my Tuesday-morning yoga class so I could get both morning swims in.

I always struggled to fit in the rest days. I fudged on that, calling my Saturday yoga class my rest day when really it was active recovery—not quite the same thing. Would I recommend that approach? It really depends on you and what your training looks like. A lot of triathletes have difficulty fitting in rest days because of the simple math involved in trying to make gains in swimming, biking, and running all at the same time. Sometimes people work out twice in the same day—a swim in the morning and a run in the afternoon, for example—so they can manage a rest day. My swim coach suggested that I could treat swimming as a rest day. Still and all, actual rest, at least on occasion, is a good thing. Even if I don't schedule rest in, something usually interrupts my ideal workout plan at least a couple of times each month.

Winter is a great time to formulate race plans for the summer. It all started with the Kincardine sign-up on New Year's Day, of course. But I had bigger plans by this point in the FB50 Challenge. With the 10K clinic well in hand, it made sense for me to do a couple of running races at that distance in April. I committed to the Run for Retina Research, a popular local race that takes place in early April, when the weather is iffy. But heck, I was feeling daring! Later in April was the Forest City Road Race, also offering the 10K distance... maybe. I could always register later if I wanted.

I set the Olympic distance in Bracebridge, Ontario, on August 9, 2014, as my FB50 goal event. The distance seemed within reach now that I knew I could swim the 1,500-metre distance and run the 10K. Despite the bike being my nemesis, I didn't actually fear being unable to complete the triathlon. I chose Bracebridge because my parents live just about an hour away from there and it would be a good opportunity to visit and get some support at the same time as I achieved my FB50 goal. I registered early to get the cheaper price. If you know what races you want to do, you can save some bucks by getting your registration in sooner rather than later. Entry fees typically increase as race day draws nearer.

I heard of a June race, just down the road in Cambridge, Ontario, that was a longer sprint distance. By definition a sprint is pretty much anything shorter than the Olympic distance. Most sprints I'd heard about were 750 metres of swimming, 20K of biking, and a 5K run. Cambridge extended it to a 750-metre swim, 30K bike ride, and 6K run.

I spent some time that winter reflecting on how far I'd come, on what I'd done and was doing that I'd never thought I'd do.

Besides riding on country roads with clipless pedals, I ran regularly, without injury, and farther than I'd ever run before. I swam with a group twice a week before sunrise. And, most astonishing of all: I started training for that Olympic distance triathlon. That's something *athletes* do, or so I'd always thought. But there I was, swimming, biking, and running my way to 50. What does that say? Well, it's either not something only athletes do, or (gasp!) I was actually becoming an athlete.

And not just any athlete: a *triathlete*.

TRACY'S TYPICAL TRAINING WEEK, SEPTEMBER 2013–FEBRUARY 2014

MONDAY	7 A.M. WEIGHT TRAINING
TUESDAY	UNTIL DECEMBER: 6:30–8 A.M. IYENGAR YOGA CLASS; FROM JANUARY ON: 6–7:30 A.M. MASTERS TRIATHLON SWIM TRAINING AT THE Y
WEDNESDAY	7 A.M. WEIGHT TRAINING; 6 P.M. RUNNING WITH THE 10K RUN CLINIC
THURSDAY	6 P.M. RUNNING WITH THE 10K RUN CLINIC
FRIDAY	6–7:30 A.M. MASTERS TRIATHLON SWIM TRAINING AT THE Y
SATURDAY	8:30 A.M. HOT YOGA OR WEIGHT TRAINING
SUNDAY	8:30 A.M. LONG RUN DAY WITH THE 10K RUN CLINIC

Tracy's Events and Milestones, September 2013–February 2014

- Started swimming with the triathlon masters group at the Y
- November 2013: Longest bike ride of my life, 50K, in tough November conditions. But I did it!
- Group run training for the 10K distance

Sam's Story: Bye Bye, Rowing and Running; Hello, Death

While the second six months of the FB50 Challenge was all about fitting it all in—rowing, biking, Aikido, CrossFit, running, and burpees!—the third six months involved saying goodbye to a new friend (rowing) and an older friend (running), though for very different reasons. Year two of the challenge, for me, was also marked by death and illness and the tricky challenge of caring for sick, older loved ones while getting enough exercise in to be able to cope with it all. There's a reason they call us 40- and 50-somethings the "sandwich generation." Between caring for needy teenagers on the one side and aging parents on the other, it can be hard to find time to sleep, let alone to work out. And of course, that's especially true for women, who as a group do a disproportionate share of childcare, eldercare, and housework. But still I got fitter, and thought lots too about life, death, and the meaning of it all.

On Saying Goodbye: Illness, Death, and Choices

Rowing got off to a glorious start that fall with my first-ever away regatta, the Five Bridges Fall Classic. So far over the summer our four-person boat had been racing 2 kilometres (a short, fast distance), though our long rows on the weekend were the length of the lake and back, about 10 kilometres. The fall though, for rowers, means the return of mid-distance, or head, races. We travelled together, we four rowers, in a very early morning drive to the performance rowing centre in St. Catharines, Ontario. This is when I learned that a lot of the work in rowing isn't about what happens that day.

But first we had to get the boats ready for travel. I got a message the night before reminding me to bring my wrench to the boathouse. My what? I was a novice rower. I don't own a wrench. What kind of wrench? I actually did have a pedal wrench but knew that probably wasn't what she meant. Mild panic ensued. I emailed back with wrench questions and got a reasonable reply: "All rowers need to have two 7/16th wrenches for derigging. I can lend you a set." I bought wrenches.

I was okay with the wrench business. Derigging boats wasn't entirely new to me, though. I'd watched Jeff get his laser (a small performance sailing boat) ready for travel numerous times. Derigging, loading, and reassembling and unloading the boats was a lot of work. About halfway through the process, I started to feel wistful for the simplicity of running. Even travelling with a bike is easier than taking a rowing shell somewhere.

The regatta itself was exciting. We had to row out to the start because the race was back down the channel. We tried to row calmly and slowly, get our strokes in order without wearing ourselves out. Doing it that way made the 5 kilometres seem endless, though. I started to get nervous about rowing that distance at a race pace. We lined up and waited for the call to start. The race seemed to be over very quickly. We put distance between us and the nearest boat, but though we got out in front, we didn't win. Masters racing involves handicapping race times based on the average age of the rowers in the boat. Our competition had snuck in a very fit 60-something.

In a regatta you need to be fast getting the boat out of the water for other boats to get in, so there was help waiting for us when we pulled up along the dock. Getting the boat out of the water and walking it back to our team's spot, about 500 metres away, was exhausting nonetheless. Our group stuck around for part of the day and enjoyed the festive atmosphere of the regatta but we left the derigging to the young folks. In the end I wasn't convinced by the ratio of rigging and organizing to actual racing. It looked fun for the younger rowers, who raced in multiple competitions and stuck around for the weekend, but I'm not sure it felt worth it to me for the one race.

I don't know, in retrospect, if that was just about rowing or about rowing in the midst of everything else that was going on in my life. That fall wasn't easy, that's for certain. My family was helping to care for my mother-in-law, Avis, who had just moved to our city after learning she had ALS. She got the diagnosis at 72, so young, and was told the disease would likely take her life within a couple of years. In the end she only lived until February, but she lived her last days with grace, acceptance, and a remarkable sense of humour, and it was wonderful to have her close by. We enjoyed a lot of family time together. The disease is sad, a tragedy, but we treasured our time with her. Starting in the fall I turned down a lot of research travel, cancelled other plans when I was able to, and started cancelling sports stuff too. You do what you have to do when family members need you. But in this case it wasn't just about duty—someone I loved was dying.

Avis and I were pretty close, contrary to almost all the stereotypes of mother-in-law/daughter-in-law relationships. Maybe it helped that I was friends first with her daughter—we were grade nine home economics partners—and so she had been in my life for a very long while. (And yes, I married the annoying older brother. That's a longer story for another time.)

Almost every time through the years when she would visit us, she'd be on some oddball stringent diet prescribed by this or that natural healer or written up in this or that life-changing book. So it's natural too that I think of her as I write this book. She was a feminist, concerned about health and wellness, spirituality, and the good life, a searcher and a seeker, and we always had lots to talk about. I think she liked having a philosopher in the family.

As you might imagine, we usually disagreed about the underlying reasons for this diet or that restriction, but since most of her diets involved eating lots of fresh fruit and vegetables, we got along just fine at mealtime. She easily fit into our vegetarian family. We did gluten-free when she visited but she died before trying the Paleo diet, at least at our house. I would complain to friends about having to hear the theory behind these various diets and how each one made her feel "better than she'd ever felt in her whole life." But as long as we stayed away from the reasons, we did okay.

The diagnosis of ALS and Avis's death made me realize that we don't have as much control over our health as we like to think. The FB50 Challenge was all about going into mid-life in good shape, and while I knew that we don't have complete control, I wanted to take charge as much as I could. There's a response to my fitness activities that's common but it makes me feel misunderstood. As we discussed in Chapter 2, I've had people say to me, "You're just going to die anyway. Why work so hard? You can't cheat death, you know."

I know, I know. I teach a philosophy course all about death. I think about mortality a lot. I know death is inevitable. And caring for Avis made it all very real.

The thing is, I'm not trying to chase off death. I'm trying to age well—to keep mobile and active in mid-life and beyond. I know I can't control everything, but I want to do as much as I can. There are many adventures ahead, I hope, and I want to be fit enough to pursue them. I love the physical activity I do now.

On the other extreme are my friends who share images of older women, typically one lifting weights and the other in a wheel-chair with the caption, "Both of these women are 74. The choice is yours to make." Having helped Avis at the end of her life, these images now make me a little angry. Yes, she was in a wheelchair, but your lifestyle and your choices don't cause ALS. Its cause isn't known. A random genetic mutation, perhaps? Doesn't matter. Eating right and moving lots won't prevent it.

There are limits to choice. We don't actually know that the woman in the wheelchair is there as a result of lifestyle choices. Not all diseases that result in one being in a wheelchair in one's 70s can be prevented. In just a couple of years, I watched my mother-in-law go from being a happy, healthy, vibrant woman who loved hiking, swimming, and cross-country skiing to being someone who needed help with basic day-to-day activities. If you saw me pushing her in a wheelchair and thought she was there because she made bad choices, you'd be wrong.

I'm all for making choices, given the context in which we find ourselves, even if that doesn't mean it's all about choice.

Come winter I started making tough athletic choices, in addition to cancelling work travel. But to be absolutely clear, these are *choices* that I made. There was no resentment, just sadness. Given the lot we had collectively been dealt, I wouldn't have had it any other way. I know lots of women who take on martyrdom for their family, but that's never been me. I'm part of a large, active family of contributing adults now, but even when the kids were little, I never parented alone. If any family is prepared to take on a crisis, we are, and for the most part I manage to feel very lucky with the people I'm surrounded by. In lighter terms, "In the event of a zombie apocalypse, I'm really grateful that this is my team."

In the midst of all of this family care, balanced with a demanding full-time job, I started thinking of some of my fitness time as selfish or self-indulgent. While it's true that caregivers need to take care of themselves, I was doing a lot more physical activity than was strictly speaking necessary from the point of view of just caring for myself.

While time for me and the activities I love mattered, especially for much-needed stress relief, I learned that some activities are better than others at fitting into a busy schedule. Come winter I made the tough decision to sit out rowing. I loved rowing but I could see that this wasn't going to be a great year for rowing for me. Unlike running and cycling, which I could fit in here and there, rowing meant making a commitment to a boat, to other people, that I wasn't able to keep. Family illness aside, it's tricky even with work travel and my duties as a sports parent. You don't just need to hold the race date—you need also to make all the training dates prior to the race.

That might just be one of the hardest things about rowing. CrossFit has lots of classes and I go three times a week when it fits. There are Aikido classes Saturday, Sunday, Monday, Tuesday, Wednesday, and Friday. Running I can do with my group that goes out three times a week or on my own. While I'm much less keen on riding on my own, I can usually round up friends to go out.

I loved rowing and I learned a lot. Certainly, it counted as achieving one of my FB50 goals: trying something new.

Running: Not Everyone's Best Friend

My next challenge came from running too much and from a small spill I took while out with our dog. In the third six-month period of the FB50 Challenge, my left knee called it quits. Running and I had to part company for a while. I had to cancel my plan to race in a duathlon and say goodbye to soccer.

Running and I aren't best friends. I knew that going in. But I like jogging with my dog. I like soccer. And I like the atmosphere at 5K races and at triathlon/duathlon events. I like taking part in these events with friends—Tracy, for example—and with family, like my daughter, Mallory, and sister-in-law Susan.

Athletic people are used to injuries, and I've had my share. I've come to think about injury and recovery as part of what it means to lead an active life. The sports medicine clinic I frequent is full of athletes of all ages. I love trying to guess which sport someone does from their injury. The last time I was there I had a bad shoulder, the result of an Aikido roll gone wrong.

One good thing about not being able to do an activity and having to do physio instead is that you have time. I'm a silver lining sort of person. Physio was also easy to fit in between work, driving teenagers places, and doing eldercare. I was still able to ride my bike, lift weights, and do Aikido, so I wasn't entirely at loose ends. I did lots and lot of glute-strengthening exercises and a bunch of stability work. Over time my knee got better—no more pain going up and down stairs—and I even made a slow return to jogging with my dog.

All good, right? Not so fast. I was on a waiting list for an MRI, but since I work at a university campus with a hospital right there, I was on their short call list. That's the list for people who can make it for a cancelled appointment in 15 minutes or less. I'd been thinking of cancelling the appointment. I'm busy and I hate to waste in-demand healthcare resources. But when the phone rang, I said I'd be there in 10 minutes. I'll run over, I said. "Really?" asked the nurse. "Is that wise?" I said I'd walk fast instead.

After a lovely afternoon snooze in the MRI (not so bad, really, when your head can stick out), I went back to work. A few days later the phone rang. It was my doctor's office and they thought I needed to come in to discuss the MRI. My doctor looked shocked when she saw me. "You're walking fine?" "Yes, why wouldn't I be?" "Well, your MRI. It's bad. Aren't you in pain?"

I should pause and say that I have a wonderful doctor. We know each other well. She likes our blog! So the frankness was just fine. She said there was "a lot going on" with my knee. It was kind of a mess. But most worrying was the "severe cartilage degradation." That sounded bad. And apparently it is—you can't grow new knee cartilage. But I was kind of fascinated by the gap between her reading of the results and my experience: I'd been jogging with my dog sometimes, doing Aikido lots, getting back to CrossFit, all without pain.

She referred to me to a knee surgeon to discuss my future and sent me back to physio. My physio dude wasn't so shocked. I showed up on his doorstep with the MRI results, wanting to know what I should stop doing in light of the results.

"Nothing," he said. "Run. Do martial arts. Ride your bike lots. Lift weights. Whatever."

He went on: "Lots of research shows it's not activity that causes cartilage degradation, and inactivity is worse for it. Keep moving."

"One thing though," he added. "Soccer. How much do you love it?"

The thing is, I played rec-league soccer for fun. I liked the teamwork and I loved the company. But I'm not good at it and it's not my favourite thing, so I agreed to part ways with soccer. Given the lack of cartilage, it was too risky—too much stopping and starting and changing directions, all hard on the knees. Good-bye, soccer.

I was fascinated by my conversation with the physio dude on the topic of his observations about MRIS. He claims that in his experience—and research backs it up—there is very little correlation between how things look on an MRI and the knee pain and immobility that patients experience. Some people have incredible pain and limited mobility but their MRI doesn't look too bad. Other people, like me, have really grim MRIS but are running and jumping without pain. He thinks that the muscles supporting the joint matter a lot, and so does activity. Again, keep on moving.

In the third six-month period of our FB50 Challenge, I also wrapped up my year-long online nutrition counselling. The program description reads, "Our coaches are part nutritionist, part scientist, part caring friend. With a little personal trainer and personal concierge built in. Together, we find what works for you, and then hold you accountable and help you be consistent. You work with a coach for 12 months, entirely online, and we ensure you get healthier, fitter and happier with your body than you ever thought possible."

I knew going in that the program wasn't a perfect fit. I took my athletic performance goals more seriously than my body composition goals. I did want to get leaner, however, even though I wasn't that focused on my appearance. By and large, I started out happy with the way I looked already. I cared much more about getting to the right weight for the race wheels on my road bike (under 170 pounds, for what it's worth) and not getting dropped on hills than I ever cared about fitting into the latest fashions or about "looking good" in a bikini, according to standards I explicitly rejected.

My reaction to my first set of bikini photos, front, back, and side view? (They had you take monthly photos.) *Wow, I look pretty good in a two-piece bathing suit for a nearly 50-year-old professor with three kids!* I was smiling in the first set and smiling in the last, and frankly, I didn't look that different. Yes, I had thick thighs (no thigh gap here—never was, never will be) and solid calves, and yes, I had belly rolls and stretch marks. But I tended to see my history written on my body through those marks and scars, which made me think about my wonderful kids and my years spent riding a bike. I felt (and feel) good even about what others see as imperfections. That fit with my general life view: the glass is always half full.

I did look different in the photos a professional photographer took at the end of the year, but hey, she was a pro. And she wasn't using my smartphone propped up on a bookshelf in timer mode.

Besides the pricey real camera, she also had makeup, talent, good lighting, flattering poses and postures, and a great attitude on her side. I highly recommend having professional photos taken as a body-affirming experience . . . but don't wait until you're thin. (In fact, don't *ever* put things off until you're thin. You might never be thin, so what? Is that so scary? Go now.)

What I liked best about the program was having access to the coaches and their support of slow, sustainable weight loss. I enjoyed a lot of the women I met through the program, too. I lost about 12 pounds over the course of the year but I also gained a bunch of new muscle. The daily readings were helpful: informative with just the right amount of research and footnotes and things to think about. I loved the emphasis on habits rather than outcomes. There was a lot of emphasis on changing your mind, with as much focus on your attitude as on your body.

I could have done without the weekly weigh-ins and measurements, and monthly photos. Again, there was lots of counselling around weighing and measuring ("You are more than just a number") but still, it felt like a bit much. I signed up for the nutrition counselling but there were also planned workouts. Instead, I stuck with the physical activities I love. I wasn't going to swap rowing, riding, Aikido, CrossFit for workouts on my own.

SAM'S TYPICAL TRAINING WEEK, SEPTEMBER 2013–FEBRUARY 2014

MONDAY	REST AND RECOVERY DAY! (BUT STILL BIKE COMMUTING AND DOG WALKING)
TUESDAY	6 A.M. CROSSFIT; 5 P.M. INDOOR OR OUTDOOR ROWING (DEPENDING ON THE SEASON)
WEDNESDAY	7 A.M. JOG WITH DOGS; 6:30–8 P.M. AIKIDO
THURSDAY	6 A.M. CROSSFIT; 5 P.M. INDOOR OR OUTDOOR ROWING (DEPENDING ON THE WEATHER)

FRIDAY   MORE DOG JOGGING OR MORE REST, DEPENDING ON THE WEEK

SATURDAY   10 A.M. AIKIDO; AFTERNOON BIKE RIDE

SUNDAY   INDOOR OR OUTDOOR ROWING IN THE MORNING; LONG AFTERNOON BIKE RIDE (RIDING ON THE TRAINER ONCE THE COLD WEATHER HIT)

PART FOUR

MAINTENANCE: Fitness into Your Future

THIRTEEN
Muscles, Strength, and Mobility

IT'S NO GOOD being able to run a marathon or ride a century on your bike if you can't touch your toes or lift your bike in the air for a photo opportunity at a town sign. Endurance is part of well-rounded fitness but it's not the whole picture. Strength and flexibility matter too, and we can lose these as we age. Women especially are at increased risk of fractures when they fall. Many women actually cite fear of falling as a reason not to get or stay active as they age. Neither of us wanted this to happen, and both of us believed in diverse measures of fitness. We incorporated ongoing training in this area into our challenge.

Women have typically associated fitness with getting smaller. For decades it's been all about aerobics or running or anything cardio, as we discussed in Chapter 11, all with the goal of losing weight and being thin. If you're a woman, the emphasis on cardio may sound familiar to you, too. Both of us rejected that picture from the start of FB50, knowing that strength training is as at least as important for women's health and fitness as cardiovascular fitness is. We each took our strength training in different directions during our FB50 Challenge. Sam pursued CrossFit and Tracy set up a home gym where she trained with body weight, dumbbells, and resistance bands. Neither of us needed to be convinced about the importance of resistance training, and we both kind of like feeling strong.

But a lot of women do need convincing. The popular imagination associates weight training with bulking up the way bodybuilders do. We've all seen photos of men and women in bodybuilding competitions, with their carved heft, literally flexing the muscles on their oiled and tanned bodies for the judges and audience. For most women, however, toned is one thing; enormous muscles that twitch and flex are quite another.

The truth is, though it's not impossible, almost no woman is going to bulk up like that just by lifting weights in the gym, even if she's lifting very heavy weights. It's not part of our genetic predisposition. Testosterone is a key factor in supporting the muscular build, and most women's testosterone levels are about 15 to 20 times lower than those of most men. That's a dramatic difference.

Resistance training benefits women in all sorts of ways, and those benefits come best for those of us who lift heavy weights. The idea that many reps, or repetitions, with light weights will get you the same benefits as fewer reps with weights that push your limits is just a mistaken attempt to make resistance training mimic cardio. That's not to say that combined cardio-resistance training approaches are a waste of time. Most gyms offer such classes. For example, BodyPump is a class that uses barbells and promises to deliver "the rep effect" and "help you achieve strength and introduce lean body muscle conditioning." Similarly, Beach Body's popular Insanity workouts focus on high-intensity body weight training that combines resistance with cardio.

But the old standby of heavy weights—multiple sets and lower reps (in the range of 5 to 8 reps rather than 10 to 15 or more)—has immense benefits for developing muscle, strength, body composition, and bone density. Stronger muscles don't have to be big and bulky. With heavy lifting, muscles are more likely to get dense and hard than anything else. When women buy into the idea that we should be focusing on cardio and avoiding resistance training, we do ourselves a huge disservice and deny ourselves an opportunity to improve our health and well-being.

In a good weight-training program, the same weight gets easier to lift over time. In order to keep the reps low, we need to add weight. That's hard evidence that we're getting stronger. Nia Shanks, whose website Lift Like a Girl encourages women to lift heavy weights, points out that weight training increases confidence. Not only do we get more comfortable in the gym using equipment that might have once seemed foreign to us, but we gain independence in our everyday lives as well. It feels good not to have to call on others to move furniture or haul groceries.

You've probably heard too that weight training helps burn fat. The reason usually cited is that it speeds up the metabolism because muscle needs more calories to sustain it than fat does. When, through weight training, your body composition changes—when you increase the amount of muscle relative to the amount of fat—the body becomes a more efficient engine for metabolizing food. That's why the Mayo Clinic recommends strength training for people who are looking to burn more calories.

You don't need to be committed to burning fat for its own sake. It's normal for women to carry more body fat than men, and you can be both fit and what some would call "fat" at the same time. Changing body composition, as opposed to focusing on weight loss, enhances athletic performance. That's another reason to include resistance training in your routine.

During the FB50 Challenge, Sam enjoyed doing CrossFit in part because there were so many women there lifting weights. Not to be confused with cross-training, which we discussed in Chapter 11 and which is about including different types of activities into your fitness program, CrossFit is an incredibly popular approach to working out with weights. It has grabbed the attention of millions, both adherents and those who watch the top CrossFitters compete in the televised CrossFit games. Combining high-intensity interval training with Olympic lifting, gymnastic moves, and bootcamp basics, CrossFit jams intense workouts into a short period of time—ideal for today's time-crunched working person. That appealed to Sam as a busy academic.

Sam also liked CrossFit because it's focused on functional fitness. It's not about what you look like—they leave that to the bodybuilders and fitness models. It's much more about lifting heavy things up from the floor without injury. CrossFit boxes (as their gyms are called) are notable for not having mirrors inside and for having lots of strong women around.

CrossFit workouts are intense. There's nothing else like them— burpees, box jumps, medicine ball throws, pull-ups, sprinting, and rowing, with some Olympic weight lifting thrown in for good measure. There's also never a dull day. The workouts change daily, and you just don't know what to expect. Also, all of the efforts can be scaled to your ability. You might not be able to do pull-ups (lots of people can't), but you can do jumping pull-ups or banded pull-ups (with a big elastic band for assistance). So there is always a place to start and there's always a place to move up to. Contrary to the popular myth, you don't need to be super fit to start Cross-Fit. You need only be ready to challenge yourself. The workouts are intense but they aren't impossible. The opportunity to measure, set targets, and achieve goals really appeals to lots of people. And it's satisfying to know that CrossFit workouts combine two things that are essential elements of good training programs: high intensity and heavy weights.

The people in the advertising images of CrossFit are almost all young and incredibly lean, muscular and ripped, non-disabled and white, of course. But the reality is quite different. At Sam's CrossFit box she found a very supportive community of real people, in a range of shapes, sizes, and ages, all aiming to get stronger, faster, fitter, and more powerful. Among the women are teachers, nurses, professors, students, derby girls, runners, rugby players, and triathletes. There are some very fit people who've been doing it for years, some brand-new people, some even new to regular exercise, and loads of people in the middle. At CrossFit, comfortable among this range of people, Sam spent a lot of time practising her deadlifts and squats.

Deadlifts and Squats: Work Your (Whole) Body

Two pillars of strength training that require heavy weights in order to be effective are deadlifts and squats. These are also routinely ignored or avoided by all but the most hardcore gym rats. Women especially avoid deadlifts and squats in their routines because, again, they require heavy lifting.

What is the deadlift? You perform a deadlift by lifting a loaded barbell off the ground from a stabilized bent-over position. The deadlift is one of the three canonical powerlifting exercises, along with the squat and the bench press. It's not exactly fun, and it is deceptively simple. People avoid it because they worry that it might strain their lower back (and it might, if done improperly).

But there are lots of good reasons to do deadlifts. For one thing, there is nothing more satisfying than being able to haul the sheer weight of a loaded barbell off the gym floor. As WikiHow says, "the deadlift is an excellent compound exercise that targets the quads, hamstrings, gluteal muscles, lower back, traps, and forearms— not to mention it will make you feel like a beast when you do it."[1]

It's also a whole-body exercise, working almost all of the major muscle groups—spinal erectors, quads, glutes, hamstrings, lower back, middle and upper trapezius, abdominals and obliques, lats, and calves. And whole-body exercises are great for developing full-body strength, especially in the core. You may worry about your back, but in the end your back will thank you for it.

Deadlifting has real functional applications, as well. Picking stuff up off the ground is something we actually do, a lot. In that sense, deadlifts mimic an everyday activity and help us to develop strength and good form for doing that activity safely.

Like the deadlift, the squat works the whole body. You can do squats with body weight, or you can amp them up with a barbell and some added weight. One of the satisfying things about both squats and deadlifts is that invoking the power of the entire body makes it possible to surprise yourself at how much you can lift.

Whole-body exercises, such as the squat, are amazingly functional. It's no good having super-strong arms and legs, exercised in isolation, if you don't have the whole-body strength to support it. People worry about hurting their backs doing squats and deadlifts, but what really hurts your back is significant strength imbalances that come from working just specific body parts. The seated bicep curl is a good example of this. How often do you sit down and lift heavy things from your waist to your shoulder? You'll end up with good-looking biceps, but unless you're a bodybuilder, there are better reasons to lift weights than that.

When lifting weights you can train for looks or for strength. Isolation exercises are the mainstay of bodybuilding, where the goal is to have a certain physique. In training for strength, you don't want to skip over whole-body movements because that's how we actually move things around in the world—with our whole bodies.

Bone Density: A Hidden Benefit of Weight Training

Now what about bone density? It can be hard to remember to care about your bones. You can't see them (no one ever compliments you on your strong bones!) and you can't even feel them. Yet bones are the frame on which the rest of your body depends. They support everything else. Bones are part of us—living things—and like the rest us, they grow and then decay. Sad truth, but there it is. Women especially have been told all of our lives that we need to keep our bones strong if we want to avoid osteoporosis as we age.

Caring about our bones, just like favouring strength over muscle definition, means turning our focus to things we can't see. How much of our focus on our health is misplaced on outer beauty when inner health and strength matters more?

The more bone density you have, the stronger your bones are. Even though genetics play a role, we can do more for our bones besides upping our calcium intake, making sure we get plenty of vitamin D and potassium, and drinking less caffeine, which interferes with vitamin D absorption (though these are important too). Increased bone density, like improved muscle strength, is another benefit of resistance training.

Once we get to our 40s, we're not going to gain bone density. But we can maintain what bone density we have. If you've not yet hit menopause and you've been skeptical about strength training for other reasons (ones we hope we have just challenged successfully above), then know this: one of the best things you can do for your physical health is to enter into menopause with good bone density.

For women, menopause causes an extreme drop in estrogen, and the greatest bone loss occurs within the first 10 years after menopause. That's why many physicians recommend that women get a bone density scan when they turn 50 or when they enter menopause, whichever comes first. That first test acts as a baseline.

Loss of bone density comes naturally with age to those who do nothing to prevent it. Exercise keeps bones strong better than anything else.

What are the best kinds of exercises to improve or maintain bone density? The best exercise for your bones is the weight-bearing kind, which forces you to work against gravity. Yep—deadlifts and squats. You definitely work against gravity when you're doing full-body weight training. Other good bets include running, walking, hiking, jogging, climbing stairs, tennis, and dancing. Examples of exercises that are not weight-bearing include swimming and bicycling. Although these activities help build and maintain strong muscles and have excellent cardiovascular benefits, they are not the best way to exercise your bones. Swim and bike, but do something else too.

Strength on its own isn't enough for our physical well-being. Flexibility and balance are two additional pillars of overall physical health. We need to counterbalance some of our resistance work, which strengthens and contracts our muscles, with stretching and lengthening, which make us more flexible, and with some balance work. We don't need to be gymnasts or pretzel-like contortionists. Adding some yoga, tai chi, or Aikido, or even just a regular stretching regime, into our routine helps us develop a different kind of strength, as well as flexibility and balance.

Yoga: The Latest Ancient Trend

Yoga has become a consumer industry all of its own, with myriad options that are difficult to navigate. Sometimes choosing between Iyengar, Ashtanga, and Kundalini, or between hot and not, is overwhelming. Not everyone has a lot of choice, of course— for you, it may just be a matter of what's available in your area. In Tracy's case, before she knew a thing about yoga, more than one person recommended a particular instructor who owned a studio within walking distance of her house. She took their advice and as a result had the good fortune of gaining a solid foundation in Iyengar yoga for over a decade. Years later, when the hot yoga trend made its way to our small city, a studio opened nearby. As a loyal Iyengar devotee and purist, she at first felt no need to try it. Then a student group she spoke at a campus event for gave her a coupon for a free introductory hot yoga class. *Why not?* she thought. And that's how she ended up trying and ultimately loving hot yoga. It feels good to "get your sweat on," as they like to say at the studio, in the hot room.

Westernized yoga has come under some criticism as an elitist activity completely divorced from its Eastern roots. Most yoga studios are far from cheap, and people pay good money for stylish, high-end brands of yoga clothing that have become the "uniform" for seasoned and aspiring yogis. It's not that you can't show up in shorts and a T-shirt, but like any activity, yoga has its own gear. And as it is with most other activities, if you don't have the gear, it's harder to feel as if you belong. The yoga studio can be an intimidating place for a newbie. Having the right mat and garb, while not required, can offer some comfort. But having to "gear up" can be a financial impediment for people. Many gyms offer yoga classes as part of the membership fee, which can be a good option for saving some money.

Some people tout yoga as a cure for all that ails us, promoting it as a means of achieving everything from increasing fertility to helping manage asthma, arthritis, heart disease, and insomnia and easing the symptoms of multiple sclerosis, post-traumatic stress disorder, emotional stress, and mental health conditions like depression. For some people, this turns out to be true, not just because of the focus required to maintain the physical poses, but also because the physical teachings—the focus of the Western practice—are just one aspect of yoga. Yoga's foundational teachings aim at the union of mind, body, and spirit. Some practices take a holistic approach based on the *Yoga Sutras,* written by Patanjali around AD 200.

Beyond all those claims, there is one certainty: yoga helps people get more flexible and more aware of our bodies and how they move, and it can improve our strength and our balance. Plus it's something that people of all abilities and ages can do.

No matter where you choose to do yoga, whether at the gym or the yoga studio or even at home, following classes on DVD or online, it's important to make sure you're working with a knowledgeable instructor. Yoga might look gentle, but some of the moves are complicated and potentially dangerous. Instructors aren't always very experienced. The amount of training teachers have varies from method to method. It's a good idea to ask questions and, when in class, to go cautiously. Not everyone has the same level of natural flexibility to start with. Some bodies do things others will never be able to do.

Aikido: Throwing Folks Around and Learning to Fall

Aikido is a beautiful, graceful martial art that's a perfect fit for women, combining self-defence with lots of balance and practice at falling. It's also filled with history and meaning. Aikido was founded in the early twentieth century by Morihei Ushiba, a Japanese martial artist who, legend has it, became disenchanted with the aggressive aspect of martial arts and developed a means of self-defence that practitioners could use to protect themselves while also protecting their attacker from injury. Aikido practitioners don't learn how to attack (kick, punch, strike)—only how to evade or diffuse an attack.

Aikido is, as martial arts go, incredibly gentle. It's a self-defence technique that works by using the energy of one's attacker and redirecting it. When Aikido is done right, your partner's movement is not forceful but it also can't be resisted (well, not without a great deal of unnecessary pain). Successfully executing an Aikido technique depends more on timing, leverage, and balance than it does strength, and often the smaller person has an advantage, making it a very useful self-defence technique for women.

It's also incredibly useful in terms of helping you fall well. Part of what makes falling so dangerous for women is that we're scared of it. The fall is made worse by our reaction. If you're scared of falling, when you do fall you stiffen up and land with a thunk. You're more likely to break something. Many seniors' fitness instructors recommend learning to fall and spending some time outside practising falling. Fear of falling keeps many people inside and less mobile and, sadly, more likely to fall when they do go out and encounter ice. Indeed, fear of falling in seniors leads to a downward spiral of more inactivity, more immobility, and more falls. In Aikido, students practise falling a lot. The most common practical use of Aikido is not self-defence—it's rolling out of a fall. You fall so many times in an Aikido class that falling becomes second nature.

Here's what one dojo says about falling: "Besides its beautiful and dynamic techniques, Aikido is known for its beautiful rolls, falls and dramatic high falls and break falls. Learning how to fall safely is one of the first valuable skills you will be taught in any of our Aikido Dojos. Safety is paramount and we teach all types of falls using safe low impact methods. We actually don't look at it as 'falling' but as 'recovery.'"[2] Of course, learning how to fall safely is an extremely valuable skill—at any age and especially as we age. Learning to fall and strength training to maintain bone strength are important fitness and safety habits for everyone, but especially for women after menopause.

Stretch It Out: Keeping It Simple for Flexibility

If you're not sure about embarking on practices like yoga and Aikido that require a lengthy commitment over time, then simple stretching could be the way to go. Maybe that sounds like an easy undertaking, but the *why, when,* and *how* of stretching are not as simple as all that.

First, the *why*. Not surprisingly, stretching can improve flexibility. It's common sense that if you're doing things like weight training that constrict and contract your muscles or things like running that repeatedly work the same muscles in the same way, it can be a benefit to counterbalance that with some stretching. Stretching is also a great antidote to the perils of prolonged sitting, something that many of us deal with in our day-to-day work lives. Tight glutes and hip flexors, lower back pain, even stiffness in the shoulders, neck, and upper back can all be alleviated with some simple stretching. A further benefit to stretching out these areas is improved posture. Stretching forces us to lengthen out of the more habitual slumped posture that so many people assume when they're leaning over their keyboards.

So let's say we all agree on the merits of stretching. *When* should we do it, then? The ubiquitous "they" used to encourage stretching before any kind of exercise. Nowadays opinion is mixed. Some argue that we should take a pass on the pre-workout stretch in its familiar held form. It doesn't prevent muscle soreness or reduce the likelihood of injuries during the workout, they say, so why bother?

Instead, wait until the muscles are warmed up, because that will be more effective in preventing injury. The post-workout stretch can help to ease the tension out of tired and tight muscles.

But not all experts even agree on that. Some sports researchers recommend to runners that, provided they are able to run without injury, they should not be stretching at all. What those researchers are mostly warning against here is what's known as *static* stretching. That's stuff like reaching for your toes or leaning up against a wall to stretch out the calves. But dynamic stretching isn't like that. This type of stretching, which includes high knee lifts and butt kicks, helps to warm you up, getting the heart rate up and the blood flowing, and focuses on improved range of motion.

Static versus dynamic stretching is clearly about the question of *how*. And as we can see, *how* depends on *when*. If when is before your workout, dynamic stretching constitutes a full-body warm-up. If it's after your workout, the body is already warmed up and a few static stretches can feel good. It's not clear whether those will do much, but doing things that feel good is a solid antidote to the perennial message that "exercise" should be a painful experience that we must endure not enjoy.

Take it away...
So many peple think of fitness as cardio, but for women entering mid-life, strength and power matter too. A good fitness program includes something for flexibility and balance as well, whether yoga, Aikido, stretching, or something else.

Try this...
If you've resisted resistance training, give it another shot. Lift all the heavy things you can, put them back down again, and repeat. Join a gym, hire a trainer, do a class, or try CrossFit. There are lots of ways to add resistance. Round out your program with something—anything—that develops balance and flexibility. Tracy likes yoga, while Sam goes for Aikido. Maybe you'll want to try aerial gymnastics, fencing, or slacklining.

FOURTEEN

Families and Fitness

FITNESS IS important for everyone, at every point in life, but lots of women with children slow down their physical activity during the years we have those children at home. Parents feel time crunched and struggle to get in enough time for their fitness pursuits. Active living for parents often competes with family time rather than being part of one big happy package. Those parents who start out with an interest in fitness really learn to excel in the sport of juggling, but children are getting left behind. Most children in North America and the United Kingdom fall far behind the recommended hours of physical activity. An inclusive approach to fitness, such as the one we advocate here, includes all generations. Physical activity matters for children and seniors, not just those in the middle years. Childhood is also the place where the physical activity gap begins, as girls get less movement than boys. That gap is made worse yet again when women devote more of our time and energy than men to caring for small children and the elderly, and thus have less time to devote to fitness activities. A feminist approach to family fitness means making fitness something we all do together at all the stages of our lives.

Fitting in fitness for kids poses a particular problem for those of us who think of exercise as separate from our regular lives, not part of our everyday life fabric. Kids then inherit the attitude of exercise as an activity to squeeze into that crammed schedule posted on the refrigerator door. We chauffeur the little ones to kiddie gyms and put them in organized sports of their own, but that can't be the whole answer. What about physical activity as part of family life? We need to start thinking about family-focused fitness and activities that include parents and children in movement. Which would you choose, running on a treadmill after your child falls asleep or running alongside your bike-riding child? As parents we're involved in developing the athletic lives of our children and play a role in guiding and shaping their choices.

Many new parents complain that they don't have time for sports or other physical activity, but for Sam, parenting and fitness go together. She still loves active outdoor adventures with her now adult children, and they've grown up seeing her roll off to work on the bike or head out to the gym while they're in swimming lessons or soccer. For years she got them to daycare in a trailer that attached to the back of her bike. Sam still vacations with her mid-20s daughter, Mallory, on cycling/camping holidays.

Sam thinks of herself as a fitness role model for her kids. They've done lots of active things together, whether it's cycling holidays, riding in the velodrome, or practising Aikido. Her outdoorsy family camps and hikes, bikes, swims, and paddles. Kids who grow up with active parents think of physical activity as a normal thing that families do together, even if they sometimes whine about it. Now that Sam's kids are almost all grown up, they still all go on hike and bike holidays together. Her youngest is the biggest team sports player in the family, involved in rugby and football, and Sam loves that he encourages her to take up women's rugby and basketball.

Finding things that kids love and that you can enjoy too is a bit of a challenge. Ditto for spouses who want to work out together. It helps if exercise, like work and school, isn't yet another thing you do apart. Finding a "together" thing may mean compromise, but that's what being in a family is all about. It's also important to think outside the traditional gender boxes when finding sports that children will love. Gender policing begins in childhood, and physical activity is the first place kids may have their identity questioned—"She's so fast. Are you sure she's a girl?" or "Boys are so competitive. They don't usually like dance classes." Sometimes, the girls want to play football and the boys want to dance.

North American kids don't do very well on the fitness front, but thinking about fitness as a family activity can help both parents and children fit movement in. According to the President's Council on Sports Nutrition and Fitness, just 1 in 3 American children is active every day. On average American children spend more than 7 hours a day in front of screens. In 2014, Canada's children got a D– in physical fitness for the third year in a row. Just 9% of Canada's children between the ages of 9 and 15 met the recommended guideline of 1 hour of activity per day. Experts blamed the dismal showing on the "protection paradox": parents try to keep children safe by not allowing them to move freely between home and school or to engage in active outdoor play, but as a result kids lead increasingly sedentary lives.

But there's not just one problem here. Really, there are at least three: sedentary lifestyles, poor physical fitness, and lack of what's called "physical literacy."

C'mon Kids, Let's Move It! Children and Inactivity

Maybe it's time we all stopped talking about children and "exercise." Our bodies, including and especially children's bodies, are made to move. We think we ought to reframe the discussion about children and physical fitness in light of the abysmal record of the under-15 set. Yes, yes, they need unsupervised, active, outdoor play. But can we stop thinking about children and *working out?* Let's ditch talk of exercise and talk instead about *daily movement.* The long-term health risks of inactivity need to figure into the story when we calculate how risky it is for our children to walk or ride their bikes to school.

It's ironic in the era of treadmill desks, standing desks, and moving meetings ("walk and talk")—when we seem to pay a lot of attention to workplace movement—that we forget about children. Yet children sit at desks for most of the day at school, they sit in front of screens a lot when they're home, and they sit in cars as their parents shuttle them hither and thither.

You might also wonder how on earth this could be true. Children seem to be leading such busy lives. Some of the common parenting discussions these days are about how overscheduled our children's days are. If you have kids, what do your family evenings look like? It seems paradoxical too that participation rates for children in some sports is up but overall physical activity is down. How is that? Two factors seem to make a difference. First, we've started to think of children's physical activity as something separate from the rest of their lives. It's that whole concept of "compartmentalized exercise." Children might, for example, play soccer but then do nothing else active the rest of the day. Children are young "sedentary athletes" (see Chapter 10).

Just how much do children sit? On average children in North America sit for more than 8 hours each day. Accelerometer results from the 2007–2009 Canadian Health Measures Survey show that the total daily sedentary time for Canadian children and youth averages 8.6 hours (507 minutes for boys, 524 minutes for girls).

Canada's kids aren't alone, if that makes you feel any better. Worldwide, today's children are less fit than their parents were at their age. An analysis of studies on millions of children around the world finds that they don't run as fast or as far as their parents did when they were young. On average, it takes children 90 seconds longer to run a mile than their counterparts 30 years ago. That was the conclusion of researchers led by the University of South Australia's Grant Tomkinson, who analyzed 50 studies on running fitness—an important measure of cardiovascular health and endurance—bringing together data from 1964 to 2010 for 25 million 9- to 17-year-olds in 28 countries. And according to the World Health Organization, 80% of young people may not be getting enough exercise.[1]

Even when children are at special classes aimed at physical activity, they aren't as active as you might think. *The New York Times* has reported on research that shows that overall, the level of physical activity in children's and teenagers' dance classes is surprisingly low.[2] On average, students spend only about one-third of their class time in moderate to vigorous physical activity. But that shouldn't be so shocking. Think about sports training—a lot of time is spent learning new techniques and listening to instructors, watching demonstrations and waiting your turn.

After sedentary living and lack of physical fitness, experts also point to children's poor "physical literacy." This includes skills such as balance and range of movement. Think of them as the building blocks of physical competence on which other skills are built. If you don't acquire some of these skills in your childhood, you're set up for a lifetime of inactive living. Dean Kriellaars is one of the leading experts in the physical literacy movement. "A child that has low physical literacy skills has low confidence to perform any activity," he says. "They have a very limited number of movements they can do well. And all of those bundled together blocks them from participating in any physical activity."[3] Many children today lack basic balance skills, for example. When you fall, you become less confident and more fearful, and thus begins a vicious cycle of inactivity that may start with teachers, parents, or peers branding certain children "clumsy." If you grow up without the basic skills needed to be active, it's harder yet again to start as an adult.

The crisis in children's physical fitness is also gendered. Fewer girls than boys get the recommended amount of daily activity, and the gender gap increases with age. Girls even sit more than boys. In the United States, physical activity among girls drops dramatically during the teen years, and many women don't do *any* by the time they reach 18 or 19, according to a study published in the *New England Journal of Medicine*. More than half of black girls and a third of white girls do no regular leisure physical activity at 16 and 17. One study estimates that young women sit or lie down for 19 hours a day, including long bouts of inactivity at school. Researchers suggested that although they might be doing enough exercise, sitting the rest of the time still has serious health consequences.[4]

Why are young girls less active than young boys? It's not a matter of natural sex differences, despite the prevailing attitudes of the twentieth century. A certain amount of risky, rambunctious play is expected of boys, even encouraged, but frowned upon in girls. Parents tend to protect daughters. But "boys will be boys," so sons run more freely.

The Play Gap?

The gender disparities that start in childhood continue into adulthood, particularly when women find themselves in relationships with the opposite sex. While women do more housework, more childcare, and more eldercare than their male partners, they get less time for physical fitness.

When we think about women's equality, we tend to focus on the big issues, on politics and economics. What percentage of CEOs are women? How many members of parliament? How much do women earn on average compared to men? Feminist writing on gender inequality shifted the focus a bit to the home, to the gendered division of work in the home, in terms of both housework and dependent care. Feminist political philosophers think this matters for both intrinsic and instrumental reasons. It's a good thing in and of itself if work in the home is shared. But there are also spillover effects: the unequal division of work in the home partially explains why women do less well in political and economic terms.

The family is also where children learn about equality and justice, and when it comes to raising and educating future citizens, justice in the home matters. So economics and politics matter, but sharing work in the home matters too. So what about physical activity? Does it matter that inequality between men and women extends to the time one has available for sports and physical leisure?

Here are some of the relevant facts: One recent study showed that people are less active in sport than they were in previous iterations of the same study, that participation rates have declined across age and gender, and that women continue to participate at much lower rates than men in every age bracket.[5] Worse still, participation rates correlate with household income. Wealthier households have higher participation rates among children and parents. The report also describes the benefits of participation in sports and these range from relaxation and fun to improved mental and physical health as well as increased life satisfaction. Lack of leisure time presents a significant barrier to taking part in sports.

Women still do the bulk of household tasks even when they work in jobs outside the home, so it's not a huge surprise that they participate in sports at roughly half the rate of their male counterparts. According to data from an ongoing National Science Foundation study, married women still do two to three times more childcare and housework than men (17 to 28 hours per week for women, versus 7 to 10 hours for men). Indeed, having a husband apparently *creates* about 7 additional weekly hours of housework for women.

It doesn't help that women often feel bad about taking time out for ourselves. Among lots of our Canadian friends, it seems as if almost nothing can get in the way of men playing weekly pick-up hockey, but women can struggle to make time for recreational soccer games. The sense of obligation can feel pretty strong. When Tracy got serious about her running training in the last year of our FB50 Challenge, her running clinic times overlapped the dinner hour on weekdays. She struggled with feelings of guilt. Every Wednesday and Thursday she said to Renald, "You can either wait for me or you're on your own." Once she got past the guilt, she managed to ask for what she truly needed: a meal on the table when she got home from her run. Renald complied, though they ate a lot of Chinese take-out that winter.

As a society, we can do things about the problem of unequal participation in sports, things like community initiatives, subsidies for sports, and increasing access to equipment and facilities. The research demonstrates that people are interested in sports and that as soon as they have enough time and money, they prioritize sports. Women place a high value on creating social bonds through sport, which should figure into strategies for public policy formation. And as a society we should be actively encouraging programs that support families in achieving their goals.

But on the family level we also need to support women in taking equal time for physical activities. Not only is it good for women's health and well-being, but it's important for children to see their mothers as physically active and competent—and for women to feel that way.

Fitting It All In: Family Time Together

Obviously, some of the issues here are big-picture and hard to tackle on your own. But here are ten suggestions for getting active together as a family:

1. Choose family-friendly gyms and fitness facilities where you can work out while your child is taking swimming lessons or other classes.

2. Take active holidays together as a family. Many such vacations, including cycling, hiking, and camping, have the advantage of being inexpensive, too.

3. Find a community of like-minded active people with children. When children are young, that might be other parents with jogging strollers or bicycle trailers. Later it might be families who cross-country ski together.

4. Just as you watch your children play sports, let your kids watch *you* sometimes. When Sam played soccer a few years back, the team had one family bring a teenager who could watch the team members' younger children. It's good for children to see their parents being active. Role models matter.

5. Be prepared for spontaneous exercise. That's an advantage of running. If you find yourself with 20 minutes to spare, head out the front door and just go. Every minute matters.

6. Make the world your gym. Take the stairs if you can, play on the monkey bars at the playground, do sit-ups with your baby, run errands on foot, and involve children in active household chores.

7. Whatever you do, don't just sit and drink coffee while your child exercises. You're at the soccer field watching practice, fine. But talk a bunch of other parents into jogging around the field. Sam watches the actual games but uses the kids' practices as a time to do her own thing (usually bike training).

8. Less desirable but sometimes necessary: Work out while the children sleep. Mornings and evenings both work and again, it doesn't need to be a two-hour event. If you've got 20 minutes and a kettlebell, use it.

9. Cultivate an active lifestyle that involves sharing the work. Even little children can help clean floors, make beds, and hang clothes on a line. When they are teenagers, don't let their activities keep you so busy that you have no time for your own. Sam was shocked and horrified to hear teenage girls complaining at CrossFit about the "crap carbohydrate" food their mothers cooked. These were the same mothers who'd driven them to the gym at 6 a.m. and who would drive them to school after. When Sam suggested that they could take over the family's meals and help out, they looked at her, aghast.

10. This will involve compromise, and maybe no one person gets to do what they love most, but try doing activities together. Whether it's martial arts or a family swim or an afternoon roller skating, make family time and fitness time one and the same.

Take it away...

Women's time for physical fitness isn't a trivial matter. Women's health and emotional well-being should get equal priority. Kids can make things tricky, but moving together as a family can make it all work and can help shift some of the statistics about all of our inactivity. It's not just about our time either. Getting support from our friends and family makes fitness fun, not work.

Try this...

Find an activity that everyone in the family can enjoy. Like the dinnertime menu, that activity doesn't have to be everyone's first-choice favourite thing. Involve your kids in watching you move and play. You have a chance to be a terrific role model. Don't make fitness something mysterious you do alone, after the rest of the family goes to sleep!

FIFTEEN

Keeping It Realistic

Achieving a Sustainable Routine

HAVE YOU ever gotten all enthusiastic about something—a diet, tennis, a new partner, Twitter—and jumped in gung ho, only to feel the initial burst of energy start to fizzle over time? It's like that saying, "Falling in love is easy; staying in love is the hard part."

And so it goes with our active lifestyles. The long haul, day in and day out, is what matters. Most of us aren't professional athletes who are paid to train in our chosen sports, with team chefs preparing nutritious meals that strike the right balance of macronutrients, and with coaches, even fans, who hold us accountable. Instead, especially for us women "of a certain age," we work, we have family commitments—from partners to children to grandchildren to aging parents—and the whole reason we want to be active is to add a dimension of enjoyment, challenge, and self-care to our lives. Adopting an attitude that will carry us through the ups, downs, and side-swipes that life presents requires some skill and good sense. That's why we're devoting this whole chapter to some reflections on how to keep it real and cultivate an attitude for a sustainable routine.

Here are some principles that we suggest as guidelines for keeping it realistic:

1. Choose things you enjoy.
2. Make it about fitness and performance, not weight loss and looking a certain way.
3. Embrace variety and try new things.
4. Make activity a part of your daily life.
5. Find a community.
6. Set goals and take the long view.
7. Develop healthy habits.
8. Focus on yourself instead of comparing yourself to others.
9. Be willing to scale back and do less.
10. When it comes to setbacks, be gentle, self-forgiving, and kind.
11. Incorporate rest and recovery into your routine.

1. Choose things you enjoy

"Choose things you enjoy" is something of a mantra for us. Seriously, we're all grown-ups now, and if we don't want to eat our peas, we don't have to eat our peas. But the invocation to do what you love might challenge those of us who feel convinced that we have an aversion to exercise.

Exercise is on many a person's list of "things I hate." We need all sorts of threats and strategies to fit it into our lives. And as we've said in earlier chapters, women are more discouraged than men in this area. With misplaced expectations about the meaning and purpose of leading a physically active life and a disproportionate focus on unattainable aesthetic results—the sculpted arms, the very lean physique—many women feel defeated before they even step foot in the gym, in the yoga studio, in the pool, or on the track.

On the blog, we've talked about the negative connotations of the word *exercise* and whether it's time to replace it with the actual names of activities we enjoy. Like "I'm going for a run," or "Heading out to the soccer pitch to kick around the ball with my friends!" or "Time for my open water swim with the triathlon club." You get the idea—lots of activity but none of it is approached with the "exercise" mindset, which calls forth images of repetitive, joyless activities performed for no reason other than that our doctor said we had to. It's more punishing still if the only reason we do it is because we think we need to lose weight. Few things make a person want to sit on the couch with a chocolate bar and bowl of potato chips more than the thought that dieting and exercise are duties they have to fulfill because they're too fat.

Author Dick Talens talks about the "myth of willpower," the idea that if we want it badly enough and have enough willpower, we will be "successful" at achieving our weight loss and fitness goals. Talens says the main reason for failure is that people don't establish a positive feedback loop. You establish a positive feedback loop when the rewards of what you're doing outweigh the pain. Willpower might get us started on a new program, but positive feedback in the form of rewards will keep us going.

This got us thinking about what would count as a sufficient reward for the positive feedback. Of course, Talens puts this in terms of results. You may need to see weight loss or longer distance or heavier weights on the barbells. But above all, you need to enjoy what you're doing. If you don't see a "return," you're not going to stick with it. He says, "Hate running? Then don't run. Don't like giving up pizza? Then figure out a way to fit it into your diet. Don't like salads? Then don't eat them."[1]

Talens argues against creating ideologies out of diet plans or workouts. If Paleo works for you, fine. But it may not work for everyone. You love running and hate swimming? Then triathlons may not be your thing, but marathons could be. This idea of the positive feedback loop is closely tied to doing what we love. It's not only about results.

Talens does his best to promote a less painful, more pleasant approach for fitness "success." But he stops short of what we'd really like to see included in the positive feedback loop. What's that? The intangible rewards.

Does your positive feedback loop include things like joy, strength, a sense of confidence, a real improvement in overall feeling of well-being? These have much less to do with the way your body looks than with your attitude toward your body. Tracy has even thought of this in terms of the way she *inhabits* her body. She now feels a sense of really living in it and owning it that she didn't feel before the challenge.

Approaching activities that have these positive effects is a form of self-nurturing. It's a whole different experience when our motive is based on needing to whip ourselves into shape because we're unacceptable as we are instead of something more positive like making the time to do things that give us joy.

Maybe you're a skeptic who thinks that there's nothing out there for you. You've tried it all, from rock climbing to rhumba, from powerlifting to water polo, and you hated every minute. We had a reader of the blog tell us that our frequent missives to "do what you love" annoyed her because she despised everything.

If you really detest everything, then we aren't really sure what to say—we both feel passionate about our chosen activities. In some rare cases, you might need to find those things that you hate the least, treating physical activity as a necessary evil with only instrumental value. But in other cases, it may just be that you haven't yet hit upon the thing you love. One of our guest bloggers is a complete convert. Rebecca Kukla talks about her transformation in a confessional post entitled, "I Was Wrong." She went from being a vocal exercise-hater to an ultra-fit competitive powerlifter and boxer.

But let's say you've literally tried everything (really? everything?) and you can't come up with something you love. If you actually don't care about your health—which is a possibility and we won't try to talk you out of it because we reject the "health imperative"—then you need read no further. But if, like most of us, you do care, then you could treat working out like medicine. You'd be in good company. Lots of people think of it in terms of "should," not "want to." Or you can do the thing that magazine articles so often recommend: incorporate exercise invisibly into your daily life. If you're mobile, park a little farther from your destination, get a dog that needs walks, take the stairs instead of the elevator, work in the garden, haul your own groceries, walk over to your co-worker's desk instead of sending her an email.

That being said, the hard-wired haters are the minority. Most of us, if we keep an open mind and keep sampling, can find something we enjoy enough to get passionate about it and want to make space for it in our lives.

And one side note about this: many women, ourselves included, have a hard time putting themselves first or giving themselves permission to pursue activities that are only for themselves. Remember that book *Meditations for Women Who Do Too Much?* It resonates because so many of us in our middle years literally do too much, and much of that "too much" is for others. Self-sacrifice is one of the "virtues" of normative femininity, after all.

We are here to tell you that not only *can* you find activities that give you joy, you are *allowed to,* and should—even if you end up loving things that sometimes take you away from your family.

2. Make it about fitness and performance, not losing weight and looking a certain way

Regardless of whether you find something you enjoy (and chances are you can and will), shifting the emphasis from weight loss or looking "healthy" or "ripped" to fitness and performance helps you stick with it. All too often, people associate being fit and healthy with being thin. But if there's any take-away message from what we've said so far, it's that you can be fit and fat, and there are lots of unfit thin people who would experience significant health improvements if they took up a regular routine of physical activity.

Focusing on weight loss, as anyone who has ever done it will tell you, is demoralizing and thankless. And it's not even the best indicator of health or fitness. Instead, maybe on your bike commute to work, you're getting there faster than you used to. That's a performance gain worth celebrating. Or you're adding more plates to the bar when you do your squats. Or maybe, though the scale hasn't budged, your body composition has changed as you develop increased lean mass.

Here's where a shift in perspective can make a world of difference. Imagine paying more attention to what your body can do than to what your body looks like. Most of us, even the beginner athletes among us, have a pretty incredible baseline. The human body is a complex and extraordinary machine that does all sorts of amazing things on the most ordinary day. Even sitting, let alone standing, walking, running, climbing, or jumping, engages muscles and requires physical effort. And what about pregnancy? Getting pregnant and giving birth are miraculous physical achievements that many women all over the world have accomplished. Where are the high-fives and kudos for that?

Taking the baseline into account, most everyone can measure her progress in relation to where she started. We can learn a lot from adopting athletic over aesthetic values. Athletes value tiny improvements in their performance, and they have to: if you watch Olympic track events, you've probably noticed that less than one second can sometimes make the difference between first place and no medal at all. Fractions of a second decide gold, silver, and bronze. Do you think those athletes and their coaches are preoccupied with how the athletes look? Not likely.

For a sustainable routine, we recommend welcoming athletic values and letting go of aesthetic values.

3. Embrace variety and try new things

Both of us like variety and are willing to try things at least once. We cross-train. Sam does cycling, CrossFit, running, yoga, rowing, and Aikido. Tracy weight trains, practises yoga, and runs, swims, and bikes as her triathlon training. And each of us stays open to trying new things, whether they be totally different, like wall climbing or obstacle races, or just different versions of what we do already, like longer bike tours, longer-distance triathlons, or different kinds of yoga.

Lots of us, especially by the time we hit our 40s, have established routines that form the rhythm of our daily lives. Routine has its merits because it gives shape to our lives and enables us to fit things into our schedules without having to think too much. But when we get too settled, it can get boring. We all know people who run the same 5K loop every day. Or they go to the Y and swim those same 40 laps, freestyle, at the same pace, three times a week. If that's what you do and you love it so much that you're still as excited to get out the door and run that path today as you were five years ago, awesome. But chances are, the routine fails to sustain you in the same way it used to.

For one thing, in order to make performance improvements, it's absolutely necessary to challenge ourselves. If we do the same thing in the same way all the time, the body adapts instead of changing. Anyone who has ever embarked on a fitness routine of any kind will know this—the same activity gets easier. And that's why variety matters. If one of the reasons for getting active is to maintain and improve fitness, then the only way to do that is to raise the stakes from time to time.

Adding variety is a great way to do that because it keeps it fresh and challenges the body in new ways. Have you ever noticed that no matter how good your physical conditioning, if you try a new activity or go back to something you've not done in recent weeks, you feel it the next day? Tracy took a few months off of yoga to make more space for triathlon training during the FB50 Challenge. When she went back to it, she did a much more basic class than she'd been in the habit of doing before, and yet the next day she felt stiff all over.

While you're working new body parts in different ways than they're used to, you're also giving other parts a break. That's the simple reasoning behind cross-training. Instead of pounding through heavy mileage every week as a runner, adding in some cycling or swimming (or both) can relieve some pressure on the body and keep you active at the same time.

The physical benefits of variety are just one reason to switch things up. Mentally, it's hard to get excited about the same old, same old. Sometimes people are committed to activities that never got them all that excited. No different from staying in an unsatisfying relationship, filling your schedule with fitness activities that you don't feel passionate about makes it impossible to explore new opportunities. You may be able to get more excited about aerial gymnastics than about the circuit of pulleys and weight machines that's been the mainstay of your time at the local gym for the past decade. Snowshoeing could just help break up the monotony of running five days a week. Paddle-boarding or kayaking in the summer could sub in for a few Pilates classes.

4. Make activity a part of your daily life

We can integrate or compartmentalize physical activity. As we discussed in Chapter 10, integrationists try to work physical activity into the fabric of their everyday lives, while compartmentalizers view physical activity as something special and different, with a sharp beginning and end time. If physical activity in your life always involves special clothes, and maybe driving someplace to start, and the activity has a sharp beginning and end time, then you're a compartmentalizer. Each approach has something to recommend it, but the integrationists have a better chance of sticking with what they're doing because their activities are literally part of their daily lives.

If you walk or ride your bike to work five days a week, that's some built-in mileage on your feet or your bike. If you're taking your dog for a walk for 45 minutes three times a day, every day, you're getting in quite a few steps. If you work on the third floor and have the option of taking the stairs instead of the elevator every time you head up to your office, that choice alone will help you develop and maintain strong legs. Everyday activity requires a certain degree of mobility that not everyone has, but for those who do, integration can be the key to keeping active in a busy life that doesn't allow for trips to the gym or long runs on Sunday mornings.

The rise in popularity of sleek and stylish fitness gadgets that people wear around the clock to track everything from their steps, distance travelled, and calories burned to their sleep patterns has an integrationist flavour to it. By now, we probably all have people in our lives who will add an additional walk around the block so they can achieve their "steps" for the day (usually 10,000, but a colleague of ours has the ambitious daily target of 20,000). And then there are the standing desks and treadmill desks. If you can't fit fitness activities into your schedule, then you can get a treadmill desk and walk all day while you're at your computer.

Some people talk about housework as physical activity. In fact, last year we encountered an initiative trying to promote the idea of "cleaning as the new cardio." One of our Fit Is a Feminist Issue regular contributors wrote a post for us, commenting on the resurgence of websites that recommend cleaning and housework as perfectly good substitutes for working out. One website says,

> Forget the gym! If women are really spending almost 2½ hours cleaning and tidying up every day, there's plenty of opportunity to get a sufficient workout without even leaving home!
>
> Housework is a great way to burn calories. But as is the case with any workout, the more effort you put in, the greater the benefit. In particular, polishing, dusting, mopping and sweeping are great for keeping arms shapely. Bending and stretching, for example, when you make the bed, wash windows or do the laundry are good for toning thighs and improving flexibility. And constantly running up and down the stairs as you tidy is a good aerobic workout.[2]

Integration is one thing. Forgoing the truly restorative potential of activity to stay home and clean the house is not a sacrifice anyone should have to make unless she is genuinely passionate about housework. There may be some who feel this way, but this kind of message seems like a shockingly suspicious strategy to relegate women into the home and the domestic duties that traditionally have been demanded of us.

That's where compartmentalizing has the edge. Dedicating time for this area of life is a way of showing self-care. It goes back to the point we made about giving ourselves permission to step away from what's expected and pursue what we enjoy. A leisurely Sunday-morning run with friends (or alone) is like a mini-vacation; it's a slice of time where no one asks anything of us other than "Is this pace okay for you?" or "Do you mind if we take a walk break?"

The best ideal is a mix of integration and compartmentalizing. Yes, incorporate some of that activity into your daily life, but not at the expense of pursuing wall climbing or aerial gymnastics or track cycling or yoga or Aikido or marathon training or swimming or, or, or... All too often many of us, as women, talk ourselves out of things that require dedicated time for ourselves. Compartmentalizing forces us to do that. And that's a good thing for us to embrace after 40 if we haven't done it already.

5. Find a community

For every activity there is a community of people who feel passionate about it. They love to welcome newbies and teach them the ways of their sport. You can find community in running clubs and clinics, triathlon clubs, cycling clubs, yoga studios, gyms, soccer leagues, baseball leagues, pick-up volleyball courts, Aikido dojos, climbing gyms, boxing clubs, rowing teams, and the list goes on. If throwing yourself in with a group of people you don't yet know is too intimidating, you can join with a friend or even pull together your own community of friends with similar interests. Find out what your friends do and, if you're intrigued, ask them if you can join with groups they're already a part of. That's why so many of Sam's friends ride—she drew them in with her enthusiasm for cycling.

Having a commitment to others is great for motivation. It's so easy to hit snooze when the alarm goes off for a 6 a.m. workout. But for most of us, when we've committed to meeting a friend at the gym or have specifically paid for coaching or personal training, chances are we'll get ourselves out of bed for it. The same holds true for the end of the work day when the choice between going home to chill or joining the club for a group run can tempt us to discount our goals. Meeting up with others can be a huge motivator because it makes us accountable. Tracy has run through two extremely harsh winters of late. If not for the running clinics she joined at the beginning of each season, she would not have maintained a regular schedule of outdoor running.

Another reason to seek community is for the infectious enthusiasm and energy that working out with others can bring. It's easy to feel intimidated or uncertain when starting something new. We don't know what we're doing, and we're tentative about whether it's going to be for us. More seasoned folks are usually excited about what they're doing and, more than that, thrilled when new people come along who want to do it too. If you've not yet drunk their Kool-Aid, they'll do what they can to get you to do just that. Veterans like to tell you all about their strategies for, say, getting faster (usually intervals of alternating between all-out bursts and then backing off to recover) and their tales of woe, like that winter they trained outside through the polar vortex.

And while there are all sorts of reasons to enjoy the inward, meditative quality of solo workouts, the camaraderie of groups can turn a gruelling or seemingly endless workout into valued social time. For example, instead of thinking of it as a long Sunday run, you may start to think of it as a different way of doing coffee time with your friends.

Working with a group can also make us work harder. Research shows that performance improves when we push harder than feels comfortable. It also shows that people who train with faster groups—not groups whose pace is totally out of reach, of course, but others who force us to push just a little bit more—makes us faster. You can get even more out of group training with a coach. A good coach knows how to put you through the paces with drills and sets that develop particular skills, for example, improved hill climbing on the bike or a more efficient swimming stroke or a better running cadence and posture.

6. Set goals and take the long view

You hear a lot of talk about setting goals. Reasonable and achievable goals can be a great motivator. Pretty much every athlete, from weekend enthusiasts to elites, has training goals. They can range from getting out to the workouts three times a week for at least 30 minutes, to increasing your distance from 5K to 10K, to increasing the weights on the bench press, to learning a new activity, and all manner of other things. Lots of women design fitness goals around weight loss. It should come as no surprise to anyone who has read this far into the book that these aren't the kind of goals we encourage you to embrace. Instead, action-oriented and performance-oriented goals are where it's at.

Both of these shift the focus away from the tired old goal of looking a certain way, which usually means losing weight and getting toned, to goals that actually improve our sense of wellness and the quality of our lives. If you want to focus on performance, you'll think about going farther, faster, longer, harder. Then break it down into mini-goals that are attainable. Maybe you can't immediately add 10 pounds to that bench press, but 5 is likely achievable. If you want to focus on action, and just getting out the door, you can have specific targets, like: *I'm going to the gym three times a week for 45 minutes to do weight training.* And it would be a good idea to have a particular weight-training program on hand so that you know what you're doing when you get there and you know exactly when you're done. This picks up on the idea of SMART goals, popular in the literature on organizational efficiency as an idea that came into prominence in the early '80s. The acronym SMART refers to goals that are specific, measurable, achievable, realistic, and time-based.[3]

Besides how effective they are for motivation, goals can make us feel good about ourselves. If you've ever set a goal and achieved it, you know what a boost that is to self-esteem. It's some kind of awesome when you can finally do that elusive headstand in yoga class. Yay for you when the day comes when you can road-bike with clipless pedals without falling over! How badass do you have to be to reach the new belt level in your chosen martial art? And please stand aside for those of us who can now run 5K when it used to seem impossible that we would ever be able to make it around the block. You have every right to high-five the nearest gym rat when you squeeze out a set of heavy squats that used to be just a dream.

Tracy can remember a time when she used to think of goals as kind of oppressive—future-oriented in a way that made it seem as if we should be unhappy with the present. In that sense, goals might seem to run contrary to acceptance, and acceptance is a good thing, isn't it? But she came around on this point as she set performance goals that motivated her to stick with her routine even on the days when she didn't feel like it. Lately, she's also found the aspirational aspect of goals to be self-affirming. Setting aspirational goals means we believe in ourselves, our abilities, and our right to pursue things that really don't do a lot for anyone else.

Goals also help us take a long view. Lots of fitness programs come into our lives through a desperate burst spurred on by self-loathing and we feel the need to see immediate results. If that's not ever been your experience, you're in a lucky minority. Taking a longer view gives us a more realistic relationship to the changes we can expect. Lasting change comes over time, not overnight. Why couple goals with the long view? We've all heard that platitude about enjoying the journey. Taking a longer view gives us time to develop a positive attitude toward our activities, maybe even to fall in love with them as they become a part of our lives. That's not to say that the destination isn't worthy in its own right, but as we like to say over and over, why not feel good about the whole trip?

7. Develop healthy habits

The most effortless way of meeting many of those goals you've set is to develop healthy habits. Habits-based programs have become popular of late because once the habit is in place, the goal takes care of itself. Let's say you want to run a faster 10K. That's a great goal. How do you get there? You can break it down into achievable action snippets and try to establish these as new habits. Maybe that means running three times a week—speed work one day, a "tempo run" at a steady pace another day, and finally a slower distance run to get comfortable with the 10K distance if you're not already there. It's kind of like if you want to write a book you need to get into the habit of churning out a few hundred words every day. With that approach, the book comes together with each daily effort. Eventually, there it is. The goal keeps us on task to entrenching the habit, and habits are useful in the service of goals.

Getting a new habit in place can start really small, and probably should. Lots of us have had the experience of going out the gate too quickly and trying to do too much too soon. If you've ever ended up hating something, that may be the reason. Inspirational writers, including Sark, who introduced the idea of micromovements as the road to realizing your dreams, and Leo Babauta of *Zen Habits*, who has written about developing habits, recommend starting "exceedingly small." Why? Because it's hard to say no to five minutes. Who doesn't have five lousy minutes? And five can build into 10, and then 20, and then the next thing you know it's just a regular part of your routine.

Another kind of habit worth cultivating is making nourishing, nutritional food choices. As you know by now, we aren't big proponents of dieting—quite the contrary because both of us have a long history of successful weight loss using diets, followed by rapid or slow regaining of the weight. Millions and millions of people are caught in this cycle. And don't get us started again on the weight loss industry!

We also reject moralizing labels like "good" and "bad" when it comes to food. It's just food. We're grown-ups. We get to eat what we want. Still and all, if you've ever had periods of time in your life when you practised healthy eating habits (including *enough* food to sustain you and your activities—we're not talking about restrictive dieting), you probably felt great. Tracy once cut out desserts and caffeine for a year—yes, that was extreme and we're not saying you need to try it. But her energy levels skyrocketed and she slept like the dead. And as much as Tracy loves french fries, which for most of her life she has claimed are her favourite food (not anymore, but she still enjoys them), she knows that if she orders fries with lunch she's going to need a nap before the end of the work day. New habit: get the salad instead. Easy, especially when it's a habit instead of an agonizing choice every time.

8. Focus on yourself instead of comparing yourself to others

How much time do you spend comparing yourself to others? And how much of that time feels good? Let's just be clear: nothing good can come out of it. It's awful at any age, but especially pernicious when we women in our middle years start comparing ourselves to the youthful ideals best left to the young (and even then, just the young with the genetic disposition to look and perform that way).

Everyone is different, so there's not a lot to be gained by comparing ourselves with others. It's tough to avoid it, though. The younger, faster, leaner, stronger women who make up the majority of the "fitspo"—also known as "fitspiration"—are meant to inspire women everywhere to aim high. But maybe you've had this experience: you're browsing the internet and you happen upon a fitspo Tumblr that combines inspirational quotes with pictures of unbelievably fit-looking young (always young! sigh) women, many in dance or yoga poses that you wouldn't be able to get yourself into no matter what body you had.

After a couple of minutes on a site like that, you might hear a voice in your head telling you that you'll never look like that (often, though not always, true) *and* that there's something lamentable about that fact (always false). Next thing you know, you feel like you're not quite up to standard.

Even those of us who are fairly reflective about these things and who explicitly, loudly, and frequently reject the idea that a particular body aesthetic is a marker of someone's worth can go into a rapid downward spiral when we start to compare.

Comparing isn't just harmful when we come out feeling worse about ourselves. It's not as if thinking ourselves better than others is a great source of self-worth either. As feminists committed to equality and to solidarity with other women, we can do better than that.

Comparing ourselves to other women can also lead to the need to compete with them. We've talked about feminism and competition. Though there is nothing inherently wrong with competition, particularly in the realm of sport, competing and needing to win in order to feel good about oneself is a pretty weak foundation on which to build a sense of self-worth.

Lots of us feel most fiercely competitive not with others but with our own past selves. When we embarked on our FB50 Challenge, we both wanted to out-do our past selves. If we can separate self-worth from athletic performance, we're on the right track. If we can pursue physical activity and improved performance because we love a good challenge, not because we think it will make us in some sense superior (either to others or even to who we are today).

You can want to out-do former selves without using past performance as a stick with which to beat yourself when you fall short of it.

A while back there was a film called *Quartet,* in which Maggie Smith plays an aging former opera star who moves into a retirement home for musicians. At the beginning of the film, she lives in the past and refuses to sing any longer because her voice is no longer what it once was. Of course, a major plot mover in the film is the question of whether she will sing again in the upcoming gala. Her constant comparison with herself at her prime keeps her from simply enjoying what she can do now. But when she compares the opera star she was in her prime to the singer she is at just shy of 80, she's comparing apples with oranges.

There are neutral ways to use comparison, especially comparison with our past performance, as a means of gathering information. But some of us are better at this neutrality than others. Here's where you need to know yourself. Tracy needs to be cautious; Sam can reflect neutrally on past performance and still feel solid with where she is no matter how it compares.

It's easy to find different ways of relating to other athletes who engage in similar activities than by comparing your performance with theirs. In this respect, comparing can have the same upside and downside as competing. Remember what Chris Evert said about good competitors? Good competitors react the same whether they win or lose. Similarly with comparing. If we can look at other women, or at ourselves at different times of life, and not feel superior, inferior, envious, etc., then we've got a solid sense of who we are and what we're about. But if looking at other women makes uncomfortable feelings bubble up in you or in some way you use it as a source of validation (or lack of it), then it may not be a healthy practice to engage in. Only you know how far you can go in this area. It's worth reflecting on your attitude. It can make the difference between sticking with it and having fun, on the one hand, or feeling discouraged and hopeless, on the other.

9. Be willing to scale back and do less

We live in a world where "Do more" is a popular mantra. But sometimes doing more is self-defeating. If you, like us, are a busy woman with commitments to family, employer, clients, relatives, volunteer positions, and whatever else, it's easy to hit a wall. Taking the all-or-nothing approach to fitness activities can set us up for failure and is a sure sign of an unsustainable routine (well, the "nothing" might be sustainable if you don't mind feeling like crap, but the "all" isn't).

In the habits section, we talked about breaking things down into small, achievable chunks. Sometimes, doing less than you think you need to do to get to where you want to go is exactly the approach to take.

One weekend Tracy had the opportunity to do an Iyengar yoga workshop with an extremely experienced senior teacher from another city. When she spoke to her about her failed attempts to get a home practice going, the teacher suggested Tracy do less than she thought she should do. "Set your timer for 20 minutes," the teacher said. "It's hard to imagine that you don't have 20 minutes." She asked if Tracy could back down from the lofty goal of one hour of practice a day and instead commit to 20 minutes a day for 30 days. Even though Tracy thought 20 minutes wasn't nearly "enough," she made and kept the commitment.

Every morning she showed up at the mat for just 20 minutes. For the first half she did whatever she felt like that day, and for the last half she did 5 minutes of headstand, 5 minutes of shoulder stand, and then added a couple of minutes of Savasana. The time flew by. Some days, she found herself wanting to do more. When that happened, she did more. By the end of the 30 days, Tracy had a solid, manageable yoga habit, and a dramatically stronger headstand.

If you're like many overachieving women, scaling back like that can make you feel as if you're setting the bar too low. But the more ambitious goals might leave you cold. They can zap the energy so much that you don't even get out of the starting gate. Whenever we've blogged about scaling back or doing less, we get a lot of comments from readers thanking us, as if they needed to hear it from someone else before they had permission.

For so many of us, our first instinct is to set unreasonable goals. But the thing is, it's actually possible to get more done with reasonable, unambitious goals.

Try working in 20-, 25-, or 30-minute chunks. The 25-minute increment comes from a wonderful time management tool called the Pomodoro Technique. Whenever you're putting off anything, you can get right back on track with Pomodoros—25-minute chunks of uninterrupted time where you're focused on one task (no email, no phone calls, no getting up, no moving to another task, just for those 25 minutes). After that, take a 5-minute break and then get right down to the next Pomodoro (which might be a new task or continuing on the same one).

If a Pomodoro is too much, you could think in terms of Sark's micromovements, first introduced in her book *Juicy Pens, Thirsty Paper.* We recommended it just a few pages ago as a great tool for getting healthy habits in place. Again, the idea is to break a project down into tiny tasks that you can complete in five minutes or less. You don't have to be a Sark fan to agree that you can do most things for five minutes. Or even less than five minutes, as Sam says in her post about the "thousand cuts fitness program."[4]

Now, it may be that five minutes isn't enough to get a lot of benefits from exercise. But on a day when you feel like doing nothing, it's something. And if you're choosing activities you enjoy, it's very likely that once you get past the initial inertia of doing nothing, five minutes isn't going to feel like enough. We have both experimented with a version of this idea where you commit to running at least a mile (or 1.6 kilometres for us!) every day for a month. If you're a runner, you know that a mile is shorter than almost any scheduled run you ever do. But it's not nothing.

The valuable idea here is that if you struggle to get motivated (you might not! Yay for you! Go do some deadlifts!), then doing some shorter-than-you-think-will-be-helpful timed sessions of uninterrupted activity might be just what you need to get the flow going again.

This is not to say we should never set big goals. We talked about the importance of goals just a few pages ago. But that's not the only way to go.

Try doing less.

10. When it comes to setbacks, be gentle, self-forgiving, and kind

When a friend has a setback, do you holler in her face and tell her she's a failure? Likely not. And yet this is the attitude so many of us take toward ourselves when things don't go as planned. Taking a more forgiving attitude to our setbacks, even seeing them as an inevitable part of the process, can help us bounce back and move on. For certain it's better than beating ourselves with a stick or deciding we're losers.

Whether something even counts as a setback is often a matter of attitude. Sure, getting injured a few days before your first marathon is a bummer. But maybe you needed the rest? And yes, 99.9% of us have experienced disappointment when stepping on the scale, not satisfied with the recommended weight loss of no more than 1 or 2 pounds per week. But if you're already feeling good about the changes you're making and your energy is up and you're learning about healthy foods while also saving money as you cook more meals at home, why focus on the scale at all?

Or maybe that deadline at work ate your workout time this week. If we can adopt an "it is what it is" attitude, that's a kinder, gentler way of accepting that it's not always going to be perfect—we're not always going to be perfect—and then taking it from here.

A key factor in dealing with the wrinkles in our smooth schedule or the slower-than-we-planned march forward to our goals is resilience.

The *Oxford English Dictionary* offers two definitions of *resilience:*

1. The ability of a substance or object to spring back into shape; elasticity.
2. The capacity to recover quickly from difficulties; toughness.

Resilience is one of those qualities that helps us wade through the muck rather than letting it stop us. We bounce back instead of spiralling down.

A training program, whether for fitness as a goal in itself or as preparation for your first 5K or your tenth triathlon or anything in between, is never just a straight trajectory of consistent wins. Some people talk about learning to live "life on life's terms." That means dealing with whatever adversity the world will dish out—the good and the not as good.

In athletic pursuits, it means handling things like injuries and illness, setbacks, the reality of our own limitations, not always performing at our best, or our home or work life encroaching on our training. It can even mean dealing with small and large disappointments, for example, the letdown when friends and family members aren't quite as excited about our passions as we are. Do you really need others to care about your 10K training plan to love it yourself?

Resilience helps reach within ourselves to find a way forward. We bounce back better when we can accept rather than resist what's happening. It's like this: if you can accept the reality of the situation first (not necessarily like it, but at least admit that it's happening), then you can always call a friend and chat about what's happening and how you feel about it. That's the social support that helps keep so many of us afloat. Talking it out also helps to give perspective.

11. Incorporate rest and recovery into your routine

With all the "eat less, move more" rhetoric, it sometimes seems as if more is always better where physical activity is concerned. But apart from the idea of doing less, celebrated a few pages ago, more is definitely not always better. Rest and recovery are both essential elements of a sustainable routine. Burnout from overtraining doesn't help anyone get closer to their goals.

In yoga, the idea of rest is built right into the sequences. No matter how vigorous and demanding a series of poses is, it always ends in the same way: with Savasana, also known as "corpse" pose. That's where you lie on your back in a neutral, comfortable position with your legs out in front and your arms relaxing beside you, eyes closed. Lots of teachers talk about "earning" your Savasana. It's a reward after hard work. It's also a way of letting the preceding work sink in. Just going, going, going all the time is not a good strategy because you don't get to enjoy the full benefit of what you just did.

The same goes for weight training. Most experts will tell you that when we lift heavy weights, we break down or tear our muscle fibres. We build muscle and increase strength not in this "tear" phase, but in the "repair" phase that follows. That means adequate rest between sessions, or at least between sessions working the same body parts. The lifting community has long sung the praises of the "split" routine, working some muscle groups one day and others the next, never the same groups two days in a row. Those doing full-body workouts need to spread them out accordingly or risk overtaxing their muscles in a way that frustrates growth.

We could add more examples but there's no need. The general point is this: We all need rest and time to recover from physical activity.

This doesn't just mean rest from physical activity. Good-quality sleep is another essential if we're going to stick to our routines. How likely is it that you'll get out of bed for a 6 a.m. swim workout if you went to bed after 11 p.m. the night before? Although it varies a bit between people and we all have that friend or relative who hardly needs any sleep (so they say), the guideline of 7 to 9 hours of uninterrupted sleep (7 to 8 if you're over 65) holds for the majority of adults who wish to be alert and healthy. Sounds as if it should be easy, but between not enough hours in a day and night sweats when we get horizontal, a good night's sleep can be elusive for women over 40.

The odd sleepless night won't ruin anyone. But a pattern of poor sleep can have an impact on our quality of life and, what's relevant here, can make it difficult to drag ourselves out the door for physical activity.

If it's just about timing, it's a good idea to make more of an effort to have a regular bedtime and a routine that slows you down at the end of the day. You know, turn off the screens, brush your teeth and wash your face, get into your PJs, turn off your smartphone and keep the screen dimmed, stop taking calls, read some fiction. These are all easy ways of prepping yourself for sleep. If there's a more persistent pattern of sleeplessness and insomnia, it may be a good idea to consult a sleep expert.

So there you have it. Those are our recommendations for keeping your routine sustainable and fun. In two words: be realistic.

Take it away...

Having the information is just part of the health and fitness story. If that were all it took, many more of us would reach a high level of fitness and stay there. Equally essential is an attitude that supports a sustainable routine. Think about which of the elements you already embrace and which you could work on. Anyone can benefit from incorporating these attitudes and strategies into their approach to fitness, but busy women in mid-life (like us) will find them especially helpful.

Try this...

Start small. Think of something you want to add to your life, whether it's yoga or a short run, and go for it—in small doses. Studies show that you get most of the health benefits of running by running just 8 kilometres a week anyway.[5]

SIXTEEN

The FB50 Challenge

The Last Six Months—
Tracy's and Sam's Stories

March to August 2014

Tracy's Story: Olympic (Distance) Dreams Come True

To say things came together for me in the last six (and a half) months of the challenge would be an understatement. My devotion to the challenge and my triathlon training kept my Olympic distance goal in a sharp focus that saw me through club workouts, two 10K races, and four triathlons in those six months leading up to my 50th birthday, from March to September 2014. These months were not without their challenges and doubts. But I showed up, suited up, and did what I came to do at each event.

March to May 2014: Spring Fever!

What a joy to see the snow melt after that polar vortex winter! The first runs in early spring 2014, when I could finally shed the hat, gloves, and jacket and step onto clear sidewalks with no fear of slipping on a patch of ice, felt like a well-earned reward. As always, we got a few false starts in March—those times when the mercury shoots up into unseasonably high temperatures only to plummet a week later, plunging us back into winds from the northwest and even snow that stays on the ground.

But by the end of March I could comfortably run the 10K distance and my swim time trials showed that I'd gotten faster in the water. My two April 10K running races showed me I could do that distance in between 1:05 and 1:10. I stuck with the 10-1 run-walk approach I'd learned in the clinic. It's a method the Running Room encourages, especially for newer runners or runners who are just trying a new distance for the first time. Whatever I was doing, it was working, at least for the swim and the run.

They say (or at least a famous fallen-from-grace cyclist once said) "It's not about the bike." But for me, any fears I've ever had about triathlon, any insecurities that could take me out of it despite how much I love the challenge and the energy of race day, have always been about the bike. But I'd gone through another winter with no bike training. If you're not familiar with cycling and triathlon, you may think that makes sense. After all, I live in Canada. Yes, there are those stalwarts who ride their fat-tired and spike-tired bikes through the winter. But you don't see pelotons of road cyclists out there once the snow sets in. Those bikes just aren't made for winter road conditions. That's when they all go inside. Yes, indoor training is a thing. And I'm not talking about spin classes at the gym. Nope. You attach your own bike to a stationary trainer and start pedalling, sometimes alone, often in a windowless basement with others. Sometimes with a cadence meter and a heart rate monitor, sometimes with a special tool called a CompuTrainer.

And what's the recommended frequency of this indoor training that I didn't do? Three times a week! Why didn't I do it? Time. I know lack of time is a popular excuse that we're told we can overcome. But the fact is, triathlon training does take a lot of time.

And in making serious gains in swimming and running, as well as keeping weight training in the mix despite the common wisdom that endurance athletes can leave it out (I disagree, especially for aging women, who are more susceptible to osteoporosis), not to mention a career, a husband, friends and family, I found my schedule squeezed from all directions. Fitting it all in is difficult. A schedule can bear only so much. That's just the truth.

Anyway, I'd fallen behind in my training for the bike. So as race season approached, practicality kicked in. Whatever else, I reasoned, at least I could *ride* the bike. Maybe not fast, but I could change the gears, use the brakes, and clip in and out without incident.

June and July 2014: Let the Season Begin— Brick by Brick, Race by Race

For Cambridge, my minimal bike training would have to do. Sam and I and our friend Chris, who had signed up to do the event with me, went out there the week before to ride the bike course so at least we'd know what to expect. I'm a big fan of familiarizing yourself with the lay of the land before an event. Most triathlons post a course map on their website and write a paragraph or two about what to expect for each portion. Cambridge promised an "out-and-back" 30-kilometre bike ride with few turns and some climbs near the beginning. But climbs at the beginning mean descents on the way back, so that evens out. And as long as the climbs weren't too long or too steep, I could handle them. A big fear of mine, that I come by honestly because it has happened to me, is grinding to a halt on a climb and being unable to unclip before toppling over. Remember: forward momentum or over you will go. So if for no other reason than to reassure myself I could do the climbs on race day, the trip to Shade's Mills Conservation Area to ride the race course a week prior was worth it. It also proved an enjoyable day with Sam and Chris.

I did not feel in peak condition for race day. I was uncharacteristically tired in the days leading up to the race, experiencing the weary, heavy-legged feeling I used to have when I had PMS. But I was fully in menopause, with no period for the past 18 months. Turned out it felt like PMS because it was! I got my period just minutes before heading down to the beach to put on my wetsuit. *Let the fun begin.*

Chris and her family met me and Renald at the park, and Sam and her partner, Jeff, were en route on their bikes, riding the Paris (Ontario) to Cambridge Rail Trail to join the cheering squad. It was a beautiful early-summer day in June, not too hot, not too humid. We got there early, so I had lots of time to set up my bike in the transition area, pick up my race kit, show up for body marking (which always makes me feel kind of badass, I know not why!), and get my head in the race. This longer distance race— 750-metre swim, 30K bike, and 6K run—felt like the big time to me after Kincardine and the Give-It-a-Tri the year before. There were lots of people who looked like serious triathletes to me, with their fancy gear, high-end bikes, and sleek, sport-specific cloth-ing. That intimidated me, but I hadn't come to win the day. I had to keep reminding myself that it wasn't about them at all. And I was accumulating my own gear anyway—my road bike, my own new wetsuit.

Coach Gabbi had given me some free advice: Try the bike around the parking lot to make sure everything is working the way it's supposed to before racking it in the transition area. I'm not sure what I would have done if everything wasn't in working order, but it was. Check. She'd also urged me to get suited up and down to the water early enough to do a warm-up swim. This last suggestion is definitely something I recommend to anyone doing a triathlon of whatever distance. For me, it gets me loosened up and relaxed, making it easier to find my rhythm. And it gets my body used to the water. Even with a wetsuit, there's an initial jolt when you enter a cold body of water.

It's common in triathlons for the swim to go out in several waves, usually by age group. You can tell the group from the colour of their swim caps. I was in the fourth and final group—the folks with the grey or greying hair under their red caps. Right before the start people always fall silent. And then the next thing you know, you're swimming.

It took me a full third of the swim course to find my rhythm, my breath, and a clear path where I wouldn't get kicked or stuck behind someone. If you go too far to the outside, you're adding distance to your swim. Everyone crowds in so they can round the cone markers as closely as possible. I started to relax into the swim as we rounded the first corner to the far side of the island we were swimming around. My breathing steadied and I felt strong and confident. By that time, I'd started passing people from the previous wave, recognizable to me from their blue caps. This bolstered my confidence even more and made it possible for me to stay calm even though there were weeds getting all caught on my face and in my hands. That would normally prompt minor hysterics because sea life in general, be it weeds or fish, throws me into a panic.

I kept my focus and made it out of the water in 17:48. Not the fastest, but by no means the slowest time. I finished in the top third of swim times overall. My swim training had paid off big time.

The bike leg was another story. I ran the 200 metres from the swim finish to the transition area with my wetsuit peeled down to my waist, as I'd been taught to do. Before jumping on the bike, I realized the air felt colder than I'd planned for, especially after emerging from the swim in wet clothes. I had to make an impromptu clothing decision, so I threw on the race T-shirt that I'd gotten when I checked in (which is really not a thing to do—you have to *earn* your right to wear the race T-shirt. But I was cold. And it was there. And the clock was ticking).

When I got to the mount line, Sam and Jeff had arrived and were cheering me on alongside Renald. I rode out of the park and onto the first climb. What had seemed so manageable the week before completely winded me on race day. The exertion of the swim? Adrenaline of the moment? Then the descent that followed scared me into hitting the brakes more than I should have.

The bike leg in a triathlon is where I have to work a mental battle not to feel totally demoralized by everyone flying past me. I continue to be in total awe at the ability of people who ride as fast as they do. Sam always tells me it's from training. Oh, right... training. Something I hadn't really done. After pretty much all the swimmers who'd been behind me blasted past me on their bikes, I stopped pushing myself. I'd wanted to finish the 30-kilometre bike leg under 1:20, and I came in just over 1:23, one of the slowest bike times in the whole roster.

The thing with being slow on the bike is that it's just that much later, and hotter, when you have to run. With the sun now high in the sky, the run would have been brutal had the route not been mostly through the woods. Still, 6K after a 750-metre swim and a 30K bike challenged my endurance. I'd never attempted a longer event in my life. My energy began to wane shortly into the run. I was still experimenting with nutrition for these longer gigs. I popped a few energy chews along the way. By the end I shuffled along and took more walk breaks than I physically needed. My mind gave out before my body, but my body wanted to tap out too. I mostly ran alone, though I kept trading places with another (younger) woman for the last half of it. At over 45 minutes, I hadn't clocked a longer 6K time in ages.

When I got to the finishing chute, Renald, Sam, Jeff, Chris, her partner and their two kids all shouted "Go, Tracy!" I know I should have felt good, but I struggled, knowing I'd come in so close to the bottom of the pack. I finished, but in my mind I didn't finish *well*. In fact, I came in six out of six in my age group and close to last place overall, with only five people finishing behind me. It would have been nice to cross the finish line before all the food was gone!

This is something you might want to think about if you're venturing into organized events but you're not especially fast: Are you competing or completing? If you're competing, who's the competition? We talk about this in the chapter on competition, but it's worth repeating here. Very few people are actually contenders, even in their age groups. So if you're competing, it will very likely be about achieving a personal record. But if the goal is to *complete,* then let that be enough. I waffle back and forth. I'll say I just want to do the thing and have fun, but then I feel almost embarrassed when I do poorly relative to others. We all have our personal demons—the tension between wanting to do better and wanting to be kind to myself is one of mine. My suggestion: If you can, know yourself, set a realistic goal, and if you aim to complete, then let yourself experience the joy of finishing.

I had to keep in mind that Cambridge was just a stop along the way to my ultimate goal in August. The next stop was Kincardine, my favourite event, in July.

My performance at Cambridge showed that even with my improved swim and running, I needed to add some more structure to my training. That's when I joined the triathlon club for the Saturday-morning "brick" workouts. A brick workout stacks the different components of the triathlon together so that training feels more like race day. With the club, we swam for about half an hour, then biked almost 40 kilometres, then did a short run to get used to that feeling of transitioning from bike to run. Consistent brick training is key to success in triathlon. It's one thing to be able to do each piece on its own, quite another to do them consecutively.

Triathlon training on the bike is a solitary affair. At club brick workouts, people got ready at their own pace as soon as we came in from the swim, and then hopped on their bikes and left. As a reluctant cyclist in the first place, I never could catch up. I had a couple of rides where someone rode with me for at least part of the way. But I hate feeling like I'm holding people back so, even though riding alone on rural roads terrifies me, I'd inevitably cut the other person loose and watched them disappear down the road ahead of me. I used those bike workouts to practise things like taking out my water bottle and drinking at speed, shifting gears to see what different gears feel like, and retrieving snacks from the little bento box I attach to the top tube of my frame.

Covering some ground on my bike on a regular basis was the only way to up my game.

If you're going to train for triathlons, you need to incorporate at least some brick training into the picture. In preparation for the Olympic distance, where I knew I'd be running at least some of the 10K at high noon, I set a standing appointment with myself that summer to suffer through bike-run workouts over lunch on hot, sunny days to acclimatize to worst-case race conditions.

A month after Cambridge I found myself driving up to Kincardine alone. All the women I'd planned to do the race with had bailed for various (legitimate) reasons. Even Renald, my one-man cheering squad, had to stay home because of work. It felt like a huge setback because having companions and support contribute so much to the joy for me. I had to accept all that and move on. But it turned out that seven women from my triathlon club had signed up for the event. And my friend Natalie, who had had to withdraw, ended up volunteering instead. When she got to the hotel, we discovered I had the room adjacent to hers.

As a reward to myself for sticking with it despite travelling solo, the night before the race I browsed the race expo after orientation at the beach and bought three things on my "new gear" list: a tri-bag for toting my stuff, reflective swim goggles, and a race belt. If you take up a new sport, you'll find that the need for gear proliferates. Triathlon gear can make brutal demands on the wallet. I'd made do with a duffle bag, but that can't compete with the dedicated triathlon bag with all of its nifty compartments. My new bag had special spots for my wetsuit, towels, my bike helmet, bike shoes, and running shoes, as well as a few other spots where I could stash nutrition, sunglasses, keys, and clean, dry clothing. It was compact and kept everything organized.

On race day, despite my having slept badly, things went well. My experience in three previous triathlons paid off. I knew exactly how to set up in the transition area. The race-day buzz energized me. I had my new one-piece "Orange Power" Balance Point Triathlon team triathlon suit on. I felt more legit. What a relief to hear that the water passed the test for the swim—unlike the pre-vious summer's duathlon, I could lead with my strongest event. A woman bagpiper led all the swimmers down to the beach playing the bagpipes. I felt choked up and stoked up all at the same time.

I had a solid performance in Kincardine in 2014. For the first time in my brief triathlon history, I made my way out of the bottom third with a time of 1:02:12, which brought me in at 92 out of 162. Woohoo! The prospect of breaking an hour one of these years gained some reality. Most important, my KWT result boosted my confidence. That surge kept me on task for the Bracebridge Olympic distance just four weeks later.

But doubt kicked in. Thoughts of *Why am I doing this?* gripped me in the weeks leading up the Olympic distance race. A mean and discouraging voice lives in my head. Maybe you've got one too. Before Bracebridge, mine came alive: *I'm wasting my time. I'm going to embarrass myself. Everyone else is going to be a serious triathlete with a cool bike. Everyone else is going to blow past me on the bike leg, and whoever doesn't will fly by me on the run. I'm going to come in last. There will be no vegan food at the finish line. My family, who is coming to cheer me on, will wonder why they bothered!* Spiral, spiral, spiral.

But this time, the counter-voice spoke louder: *This is the day I've trained for all year, the culminating moment of the FB50 Challenge! Mum, Dad, and Renald are all coming! No matter what happens, I'll finish! And it'll be fun. And maybe, just maybe, I'll cross the finish line before they finish the pizza.*

On that clear, hot, sunny day, not the least bit humid, Renald and I made it to Annie Williams Memorial Park, a grass-covered picnic area on the river, before 7 a.m. My nerves settled into my stomach halfway there, and I had to run from the car to the bathroom before I could even think of getting my stuff ready or checking in.

By the time I got back, Renald, my one-man pit crew, had my bike unpacked and my bag ready to go. I pumped up my tires—a well-formed habit I've gotten into doing before every single time I take the road bike out. I grabbed my bag and wheeled the bike

down to the registration area where I picked up my bib—#335—
and my T-shirt. (I should have signed up for the cap—it's always
a toss-up when you have to choose months before.)

As I entered the transition area, I heard someone calling my
name. I turned around to see one of the guys from Balance Point
Triathlon, the club I swam with through the winter and joined
for the summer. My club suit made it easy for him to pick me out
of the crowd, and his club suit made it easy for me to recognize
him. It felt good to have someone acknowledge my understand-
able nerves and assure me that I'd be fine.

I'd driven the bike course the day before. I would have liked
to have ridden it, but it didn't seem like a wise thing to do within
less than 24 hours of the race. The hilly course has lots of different kinds of ascents and descents—from short and steep to slow
and steady. I'd gotten over my terror of hills, no longer regarding
them with complete dread. But the course did kind of scare me.

I set up my transition area in the way I've become accustomed
to, laying everything out on my navy blue towel, folded in half
beside my bike.

I rested my wetsuit over my racked bike and went out to chat
with Renald. The announcer kept reminding us there would be
a pre-race meeting near the water at 8 a.m. to explain the "time
trial start" for the swim. The narrow course on the river made the
usual group start from the beach impossible. Instead, we would
go one at a time, in five-second intervals, in order of our bib numbers (assigned by age).

With about five minutes to go until the meeting, I slicked
myself up at key points with Body Glide and wriggled into my
wetsuit, up to my waist.

Athletes were already in the water doing swim warm-ups. My
parents arrived, lawn chairs in hand. Renald set them up in a
prime location at the swim finish while I dashed off to the meeting.

For the time trial start we would line up on the dock and then
in the water, 50 at a time, when the announcer called our group.
All that waiting around after the race has begun makes it more
nerve-racking than the typical "wave" start from the beach.

The fastest athletes—the elites competing in the Ontario championships and seeking a spot on the Canadian national team—swam first, then the age groups from youngest to oldest.

Since my group wouldn't be called for about 15 more minutes after the start, I waded into the river for a practice swim. The oozy, soft bottom squelched between my toes, which I couldn't see through the dark, briny water. Not my favourite conditions, but the warmer water meant no alarming jolt when it filled the wetsuit and no problem for the face, hands, and feet.

I hung with Renald and my parents for a few minutes but then felt like I really needed to get my head in the game. Moving closer to the dock, I heard my name again and turned around to encounter a colleague from the university's medical school. He'd done the course a few times, and started talking about the bike course. As soon as he began to describe the steep hill just a few kilometres from the start, at Santa's Village, I felt my stomach drop a bit.

Then they announced my group.

The Swim: 1.5 Kilometres

By the time I got to the front of the line I didn't have a lot a time to think. *Five, four, three, two, one.* I settled into pace after about 50 metres. For the first time in my race history, I had no trouble establishing my rhythm and my breathing at the beginning of a race. I passed a few people right away.

The swim took us along the shoreline on one side of the river for 720 metres, then we crossed to the other side (about 10 metres) and swam back, down along the other shore to the finish. I sighted regularly, keeping the enormous orange markers in view and on my left. Green cones marked the three turns. The first one took forever to come into view. I picked up the pace when I rounded it—I had plenty in the tank for a negative split on the swim. I got caught behind someone on that stretch, having to hold up so as not to get kicked in the face, but I altered my course slightly to find a clear path. I glimpsed some gnarly tree branches under the water, which freaked me out (again: irrational fear of things in the water).

I sighted the final green marker at the end of the swim, indicating the last turn which would be followed by a short stretch to the shore and the run up to the transition. I gunned it.

On shore, Mum, Dad and Renald were yelling "Go, Tracy!" I smiled, reached around to unzip my wetsuit, and ran a bit faster.

Swim time: 33:45 minutes

Transition 1

I got all flustered in the transition area, despite having mapped out my course visually from the entrance prior to the race. I had to double back out of the duathlon bike area, and when I found my bike, I looked at everything on my towel and for a brief moment had no idea what to do next. *Okay. Regroup.* I pulled off the wetsuit and dabbed myself off with a towel. On a hot day, it hardly matters if you're still wet.

I just wanted dry feet. So I threw the towel down and stepped on it while I grabbed my socks and pulled them on. Then the glasses and the helmet, bike shoes, gloves. Things moved in slow motion (not the best thing for a race). I unracked the bike and ran under the "bike out" arch to the mount line.

"Come on, Trace!" Mum shouted.

T1 time: My T1 was my slowest ever, somewhere in the 3 minute range.

The Bike: 40 Kilometres

Here's the part where everyone passes me.

But I knew that would happen, so I had my own modest goals for the bike. The plan: Use it to build confidence on my ability to make it up hills, fearlessness in letting it fly on the descents, and awareness of cadence and the sensation of "spinning" the pedals, especially the part where you're supposed to feel like you're scraping mud off your shoes.

The sun blasted down from high in the sky by this point. And 40 kilometres is kind of far.

But there were some highlights along the way. I *did* make it up all those challenging hills. That Santa's Village hill my colleague told me about defeated at least one person in front of me—he was picking himself up after he had fallen over trying to make it. Me? I had to grind my way up, huffing and puffing all the way, a long, steady climb that went on and on and on just before the turnaround got me into positive self-talk mode. I reminded myself that cycling types always tell me I'm built to be a climber because I'm small. I repeated, aloud, "I'm a climber, I'm a climber, I'm a climber, I can do this, I can do this." And I used all the tips from Sam's cycling coach, Chris, who Gabbi had called in to the club for a hill-climbing workshop. I let up a bit as I came into a hill, then spun at a high cadence into the climb, doing that mud scraping thing.

It's tough to eat and drink on the bike, but I needed to do both if I didn't want to suffer dehydration and a depleted energy store on the run. I had some homemade endurance gel shot blocks handy in my new and wonderful bike bento box. I popped them at regular intervals and drank my water, laced with Emergen-C on the flats. I practised drinking while pedalling. But each time I drank I lost time.

The ride had its downsides too, of course—that demoralizing feeling I felt when everyone left me in the dust. Other than that guy who fell over and another poor soul who had a flat, I didn't pass anyone on the bike ride. But oh, did people pass me! Each time, I had to buck myself up with some positive self-talk and remind myself that my only goal was to complete the race. When I turned around, I saw a tiny handful of people behind me. But yeah, it's frustrating not to know what to do to go faster. After the race I spoke to a woman who was the first person I've ever talked to who "got it." She too said that she just doesn't understand how people go faster on the bike. It seemed impossible to her that her time would ever improve. Well, that's how it seemed (and seems) to me. What do I recommend as an antidote to this feeling? Training. I've never committed fully enough to making progress on the bike.

Then there was that last lonely leg of the bike, when I could see no one else and I still had a 10K run ahead of me and the position of the sun said almost high noon and I knew I'd been out there on the bike longer than I'd planned—right then I considered bailing and downgrading my September triathlon at Lakeside to a sprint distance. But the blog forces public accountability. And that can really motivate a person. So despite that little melodrama in my head, I persevered (*"I'm a climber, I can do this"*).

When I got off my bike at the dismount line, Mum said, "Wow, you look fresh!"

Bike time: 1:55:17 (I had hoped for between 1:30 and 1:45.)

Transition 2

Uneventful except that the last thing I wanted to do at that point was to run a 10K.

T2 time: Under 1:30

The Run: 10K

Maybe I looked fresh, but I felt like I wanted to lie down on the cool grass in the shade of an old maple tree beside the river. I embraced a simple strategy: I would try to keep my pace between 6:30 and 7:00 per kilometre, and that would bring me into the finish line within 1 hour and 10 minutes. I knew I could *complete* the 10K, but could I maintain a decent pace?

Not quite. The flat course had few shady bits, and the heat of the day bore down on me. At the water stations, I took extra to pour over my head. That refreshed me for a few seconds each time.

Ignoring the received wisdom never to try anything on race day you've not tried before, with 5K left to go, I drank some Hammer HEED for electrolyte replacement. Mistake. Within minutes, I felt bloated and heavy. And overheated. And tired.

On an out-and-back course, the people heading back shout out much-needed words of encouragement to the slower athletes. This race series has the added bonus of putting our first names in large letters on the bibs, so people could support one another by name. It helps.

I passed no one. And by then, there weren't many people left to pass me either. So I ran alone.

252 FIT AT MID-LIFE

After the turnaround, about 10 cups of water over the head later, I noticed for the first time that my shoes were saturated with water. Each time I'd dumped it over the front of my head, it had made its way down to my shoes. Slosh, slosh, slosh. That was for the last 4K.

Running lacks the fear factor. In the worst-case scenario, you walk. Nothing dangerous about it, you just slow down. I felt my pace faltering. I started to play little games with myself about making it to that tree or that house or that water station or that distance mark.

A guy named John passed me at the 8K mark, with the words, "I wish that said 9K." I kept him in sight the rest of the way but couldn't keep up.

Finally, I turned into the park again. I wanted to fly down the grassy slope to the finish line but my body would only jog. Mum and Dad and Renald hollered out, "Go, Tracy!" and others chimed in with "You're there!"

Run time: 1:18:48

Race time: 3:52:36

The Finish Line

Of the 348 who finished, I placed at 343. Six others succumbed to the heat and didn't make it to the end. My family greeted me at the finish line, Mum moved to tears by my accomplishment, Renald close behind her.

I did it! It took a bit for it to sink in. I soaked in the moment I'd been training for all year. My Fittest by 50 goal, accomplished! If you want to feel a sense of humble achievement, finish in the bottom 10. Those of us who endure to the end are out there a long time. Sean Bechtel, the champion, finished the entire course almost two full hours ahead of me in an astonishing 1:55:19.

The thing we most miss out on, us in the bottom ten, is the energy of the crowd. By the time I got there, everyone had pretty much dispersed. A few people still hung around eating pizza and packing up their stuff, but put it this way: before I left the volunteers' pizzas arrived. We don't get to feel the excitement of the announcer and people cheering at the finish line and coming in with other competitors. It's there in the shorter races—I felt it in Kincardine. I love that finish-line feeling you can only get from having enough people around to create that buzz in the air.

Never mind. I did it. And in every picture of that day I'm smiling. FB50 mission accomplished!

I squeezed two more big adventures in before my 50th birthday in late September 2014. Renald and I rented an RV and saw the Grand Canyon before attending Burning Man, an indescribable experiment in temporary community, held at the end of August every year in the Nevada desert. And ten days after we got back, on a cold September Sunday, I completed the Lakeside Olympic distance triathlon, shaving a few minutes off of my Bracebridge time.

TRACY'S TYPICAL TRAINING WEEK, MARCH–SEPTEMBER 2014

MONDAY	7 A.M. WEIGHT TRAINING
TUESDAY	UNTIL JULY: 6–7:30 A.M. MASTERS TRIATHLON SWIM TRAINING AT THE Y; FROM JULY ON: 6 A.M. OPEN WATER SWIMMING WITH THE TRIATHLON CLUB
WEDNESDAY	7 A.M. WEIGHT TRAINING (ON HOT DAYS, NOONTIME BIKE-RUN BRICK IN ANTICIPATION OF GOAL EVENT CONDITIONS)
THURSDAY	7 A.M. RUNNING
FRIDAY	6 A.M. OPEN WATER SWIMMING WITH THE TRIATHLON CLUB
SATURDAY	8:30 A.M. OUTDOOR SWIM-BIKE-RUN BRICK WORKOUTS WITH THE TRIATHLON CLUB
SUNDAY	8:30 A.M. LONG RUN WITH THE RUN CLUB

Tracy's Events and Milestones, March–September 2014

- April 2014 Run for Retina 10K, London, Ontario
- April 2014 Forest City Road Race 10K, London, Ontario
- June 2014 Cambridge Sprint Triathlon, Cambridge, Ontario
- July 2014 Kincardine Women's Triathlon, Kincardine, Ontario
- August 2014 Bracebridge Olympic Distance Triathlon, Bracebridge, Ontario
- September 2014 Lakeside Olympic Distance Triathlon, Lakeside, Ontario
- Bonus points: After the FB50 Challenge and because of her FB50 training, Tracy ran her first half marathon in October 2014 (Toronto) and a week later achieved a personal best in the Halloween Haunting 10K, dressed as a witch.

Sam's Story: Sam's Life of Riding

I started the FB50 Challenge by branching out from the bike—picking up running and rowing and CrossFit—but on the home stretch I realized it's okay to love one thing the most and I came home to cycling, but stronger and faster. I started taking cycling all the more seriously, hiring a cycling coach and setting myself some big goals. In July 2014, the second-last month of the challenge, I logged some 1,300 kilometres on my bike. I'd enjoyed my time away from the bike, but I was also very happy to come home.

Thanks to my cycling coach, I had my initial fitness tested—max heart rate and vo_2 max—and I started wearing a heart rate monitor again when training on the bike. I took up structured workouts with time in various heart rate zones. It's fun to watch improvement in heart rate recovery as you get faster and stronger on the bike. I had a good amount of base fitness going in, but the specialized bike workouts were new. I started riding with faster people, and the range of speeds at which I could comfortably ride grew.

My interests weren't only in racing, which was a good thing. As I age, I'm finding it much harder to find people to race against.

But I like riding fast, riding long distances, and being able to keep up with people with good bike skills, the kind of people who ride in close formation and take turns at the front going into the wind, the kind of people who race up hills and go fast coming down on the other side. While I planned to get back into bike racing as part of the FB50 Challenge, I had to readjust my expectations. Unlike running, which has seen a boom in amateur racing, that hasn't really happened for cycling. There's too much skill involved, maybe, and too much danger riding fast in groups. I'm not sure why, honestly. Lots of my women riding friends have given up racing, though there seems to be no shortage of 50-year-old men out there. Although at the end of the first year of the challenge, along with two thousand other riders, I took part in the Niagara Falls Gran Fondo. Part ride, part race, it marked my return into bike-racing culture.

People often ask how long I've been a cyclist. That's a tough question to answer. Like many people, I rode a bike as kid. It was the 1970s, so my bike was purple and had a banana seat, a backrest—also known as a "sissy bar"—and funky handlebars with plastic streamers. But come high school, I was too cool for a bike. Driving seemed glamorous back then, not costly and environmentally unfriendly. It wasn't until university that I caught the bug again. And the Raleigh hybrid I bought in Halifax saw me through grad school in Chicago, where I fell in love with the city's lakeside bike paths.

I commuted by bike for years, through some of undergrad, grad school, and as a tenure-track faculty member. When I started running, as I approached 40, road-cycling academic colleagues joked that it was time I got a "real bike."

When running led to triathlon, I did just that. It turned out I was a much faster cyclist than a runner from the very first time out. I was surprised to find myself passing many of the people from my triathlon clinic, people I rarely saw when we were out there running, they were so far ahead. What I hadn't realized is that I'd been "training" for years, riding a bike to and from work, and later towing a trailer full of babies and toddlers. "Go faster,

Mum, go faster!" In fact, we'd rented a family cottage one holiday right on the route of the Kincardine Women's Triathlon that Tracy and I did as part of the FB50. So the first time I encountered that rise from the beach road to the town road was with two toddlers in the bike trailer.

And so when running injuries took me out of triathlon, I kept riding. I started riding with a local bike club and on several sabbaticals in Australia and New Zealand. I trained regularly with a racing club and discovered the world of road racing, time trials, and criteriums. I also spent some time on the boards of our local velodrome, riding a fixed gear, no brakes track bike over the winter. Cycling was and is a huge part of my life. I take cycling holidays, ride with friends, commute by bike, and would love to race more.

Starting with the cycling coach meant taking it all a bit more seriously. The cycling coach's regimen required something new of me, riding my bike indoors on a trainer through the winter. That last winter of the FB50 Challenge I started lugging my bike and a trainer in the trunk of my car to Coach Chris's basement, where I rode indoors—tracking heart rate and cadence, doing sprint drills, and sustained efforts—going nowhere! It doesn't matter that we listened to fun music and worked hard together, riding on a trainer for 90 minutes at a time is tough—physiologically and physically demanding. I like being outside, and in the winter I typically switch to running, skating, and cross-country skiing. Coaching wisdom though is that while cross-training can be a good thing to avoid burnout, the only way to improve your performance on the bike is to train on the bike.

Indoor cycling through the winter meant come spring I was in pretty good shape. No more spending the first month getting my cycling mojo back. We started riding outside earlier than I was used to, in the cold months of March and April. Again, it meant admitting I was taking my riding seriously, because lots of the training wasn't fun. Lance Armstrong says of the suffering while riding a bike that he doesn't do it in spite of the suffering; he does it because of the suffering: "Once, someone asked me what pleasure I took in riding for so long. 'PLEASURE????' I said. 'I don't understand the question.' I didn't do it for the pleasure; I did it for the pain." For good or bad, I'm no Lance, but I did come to improve my ability to suffer on the bike that year.

Riding for Smiles and Scenery

But biking isn't all about suffering. Come June I did a self-supported biking tour of Manitoulin Island with my life partner, Jeff. We had a great time cycling there—on the world's largest island in a freshwater body of water—and we're planning a return journey, next time with a bigger group of friends and family. The country roads were just about perfect: rolling hills, no traffic, and lots of great views. There was a lot of wildlife, too. On the road it was deer and turtles mostly, though we did have one very free-range hen run across the road in front of us. The island also has a rich history that we had time to learn about as we travelled around, including lots of First Nations history and culture.

I love cycling holidays. I find riding a bike the perfect speed at which to see a new place, and I love the combination of riding and sightseeing. The terrific thing about doing one after a winter of riding indoors is that I could focus on the places and the journey. We left Lance's philosophy behind on this holiday and enjoyed ourselves.

The challenge with riding independently is that our nice road bikes weren't great for carrying stuff. Yet on a multiday outing, they're the bikes we want. After looking around and reading online, we bought a trailer big enough to hold our gear for a week-long cycling adventure. We stayed in B&Bs and motels, no camping, so we packed a few changes of clothes each, planning to do laundry en route, as well as snacks, sunscreen, bike tools, spare tubes, and tires—and off we went.

We drove to Tobermory and stayed in the Blue Bay Motel before catching the mid-morning ferry to Manitoulin. The MS *Chi-Cheemaun* doesn't require reservations for bikes and you get to board the ferry first—bikes, motorbikes, cars, then motor homes, trucks, and other vehicles.

The bike holiday was a terrific way to get in shape for the cycling season and get lots of very pleasant kilometres in on the bike. But my next summer biking adventure was a little harder and more adventurous.

Sam Rides for Life

For years I've been intrigued by the Friends for Life Bike Rally, a six-day charity ride from Toronto to Montreal. It's the main fundraiser for the Toronto People with AIDS Foundation, and it's a big commitment. I decided to make the bike rally the culminating event of my FB50 Challenge. It's a 660-kilometre ride, over six days, camping along the way. When readers of our blog found out I'd done the rally, they asked two questions: How tough was it? Could they do it? Here's my answer to the first: It was tough. It rained four out of the six days, including, on our first night, an incredible overnight thunderstorm that blew people's tents off the ground. How hard? Harder than childbirth, say? Our team co-captain Stephanie Pearl-McPhee said she felt it was harder than childbirth or any parenting crisis she's come across, partly because it was optional:

Childbirth might be hard, but really, you don't have any choice. Once you're pregnant, there's only one why [*sic*] that it can end. Somehow, some way, a baby is going to come out of your body, and no matter how it does that, you're in it. There's no way out. You can cry and be afraid and it can be hard, but it's going to happen to you anyway, whether you're brave or not. Parenting? Illness, crisis? Same deal. You're in it, and nobody rides by in a car while you're trying to deal with it all and asks if you'd like a ride past all the hard bits. You've got to do it, and you do. We all do, somehow.[1]

Personally the riding on any one day wasn't challenging. I regularly ride more than 100 kilometres in a day. And I've been riding long distances with groups for a while. But the accumulation of those days is what makes it tough. Also, the second day in the rain and wind would have been tough on its own. Wind, rain, cold—not to mention starting wet and cold with very little sleep after the thunderstorm the night before. But it was also really wonderful in ways I hadn't expected. I really liked getting to know people over the course of the rally. I liked riding with different people on different days, some fast, some slow, some chatty, others not.

That's the nice thing: you're not doing it alone. There are almost as many crew as riders. They're involved in planning and preparing food, transporting gear, setting up each new site, route management, road safety, bike fixing, and more. Oh, and giving massages. I loved that part especially. There's a very strong team atmosphere that's part of the bike rally. I thought our team co-captains did an amazing job.

Stephanie:

Riding your bike to Montreal does nothing to help sick people. Nothing. You could do it a hundred times, and without the support of people like all of you who donated, it wouldn't change one little thing about the world, or the way it can be for people who are suffering. It is what all of you have done—your generosity, that turns the action we're all undertaking into real change. Real kindness. Real love.[2]

My team raised over $150,000. The rally as a whole raised more than a million dollars. I was very happy to have chosen to mark my 50th birthday by contributing to this beautiful effort.

Now the next question: Could you do it?

Sure. Buy a bike if you don't own one, start training now if cycling is new to you, follow the spring training plan, and you'll be fine. I actually think that most people could do the distances required by the rally. There are morning and afternoon breaks, and people ride at a wide range of speeds. Training well, though, means you can ride faster, get to camp earlier, and feel strong the next day. I was happy with the effects of all the bike riding I'd done in advance. Most days I arrived at camp mid-afternoon thinking I could have ridden a bit more if need be. And I woke up each morning ready to ride again, not sore.

Different people find different aspects of an event like this challenging, other than the riding. I love camping, think the indoors is overrated, and own some pretty nice camping gear. I sleep happily and well in a tent, and when I'm tired, noise doesn't bother me much. But I got the sense that not everyone shared my love of the great outdoors. One friend who did the rally in years past said he found the social demands challenging. It was too much like summer camp, he thought. Well, I'm a nerdy professor and spent time alone with books quite happily and no one dragged me out of my tent.

Now, another friend who loved that aspect of it said it was like the queer summer camp he never had as a kid. That made me smile. I'd say the sexual orientations of the rally participants, riders, and crew were all over the spectrum. If you're curious, there were quite a few opposite-sex couples. But it was a totally lovely experience for me, as a bisexual, to be in a place where the majority of people were gay and assumptions weren't made about sexual orientation on the basis of the relationships you're currently in.

A non-cycling-related surprise also happened at the end of the challenge. While I'd given up the extra activities I'd taken on, I continued to practice Aikido. And soon after our FB50 Challenge ended I tested for another Aikido belt, surpassing my Aikido-related goals.

In the end, my fitness plans in the second year of the FB50 Challenge were thrown off the rails by some major life events. I'd made plans to celebrate my 50th birthday with a big kickass party. I planned to focus on fitness, to give 50 a swift kick in the pants, to run away really fast from 50, to lift 50 up over my head a dozen times, and keep on moving.

Instead, the second year of our challenge had other plans. First there was the death of my mother-in-law from ALS. Then, just months after her death, my father-in-law also died, in the middle of the final summer of our fitness challenge. His death was the opposite sort of death. It was sudden and peaceful, and came out of the blue—he died of a stroke. Again, we made plans to travel, planned memorial services, sorted through belongings, made calls, hugged and cried a lot, and told stories. I still miss both of my parents-in-law. And frankly, I'm still shocked some days they're not here.

It had been a really rough few years. Truth be told, if the final year of the FB50 Challenge were to be defined by a singular focus it would be Family not Fitness, and Death rather than Athletic Achievement. But the bright side, from the perspective of fitness, is that my athletic activities, rather than always competing for time and attention, actually helped me get through some super tough times. There was solace and comfort to be found on my bike, or walking through the woods with dogs, I also had the energy to help others and to reach out and make the world a bit better through the Friends for Life Bike Rally.

What started out as a personal, maybe even slightly selfish, thing—focusing on my own physical fitness—ended up being the thing that helped me help others. Without the challenge project, without Tracy's friendship, without the blog, I might have easily abandoned physical activity and wallowed in sadness. Instead, the regular fitness activities and the community the blog provided helped me make it through a couple of very hard years. By the end of the challenge I felt I'd become a better person—not just fitter and faster one, but also more connected to friends, to family, and to the larger community.

SAM'S TYPICAL TRAINING WEEK, MARCH–SEPTEMBER 2014

MONDAY	**7 A.M. CROSSFIT;**
	7 P.M. AIKIDO
TUESDAY	**6 A.M. CROSSFIT;**
	5 P.M. INDOOR BIKE TRAINER CLASS
	(OR OUTDOOR RIDING)

WEDNESDAY	6:30 P.M. AIKIDO
THURSDAY	6 A.M. CROSSFIT; 5 P.M. INDOOR BIKE TRAINER CLASS (OUTDOOR STARTING IN MARCH)
FRIDAY	REST UP FOR THE WEEKEND
SATURDAY	AIKIDO IN THE MORNING UNTIL THE WEATHER PERKED UP, THEN OUTDOORS BIKE RIDING
SUNDAY	BIKE RIDING OR RUNNING, WEATHER DEPENDING; EVENING, HOT YOGA

Sam's Events and Milestones, March–September 2014

- April 2014 Run for Retina 5K, London, Ontario
- June 2014 400 km cycling holiday, Manitoulin Island, Ontario
- July 2014 Friends for Life Bike Rally, 600 km from Toronto to Montreal to raise money for the Toronto People with AIDS Foundation
- September 2014 The Halton Epic Tour (Toronto Gran Fondo), 80 km
- BONUS POINTS: After the FB50 Challenge, because of her training during the challenge, Samantha successfully tested for 4th Kyu, full green belt, in Aikido, November 2014.

Epilogue

Life after 50 and Reflections on the FB50 Challenge

Tracy on Turning 50: Reflections on the FB50 Challenge

The thing with challenges is that lots of people hit their goal and then come to a screeching halt. That's not my style. My 50th birthday, with a fantastic cake party, was just a day. I'd met my fitness goals, completing the events I'd planned for. But I didn't feel as if I was "finished." I may have been fitter than ever before in so many ways, but I hadn't hit my peak.

A month after I turned 50, I did my first half marathon. Two weeks after that, dressed as a witch at the Halloween Haunting, I ran a personal-best 10K. Then it was time to settle in for the winter. I finally did that indoor bike training everyone always talked about. I also signed up for my two longest running events ever: the Around the Bay 30K (locally known as ABT) in Hamilton (March 29, 2015) and the Mississauga Marathon five weeks later, my first full-length marathon. A training clinic geared at the ABT kept me going through the tough winter. I completed both events. Yes, I did!

I don't spend a lot of time thinking about my age. Being so early into a new decade is kind of liberating. Like I get to enjoy "the youth of old age" for a long time before another "big birthday" comes my way. And enjoy it I am. The Kincardine Women's

Triathlon remains my favourite event. In July 2015, Samantha and I were part of a group of nine women who went to Kincardine together to do the race. Some of the women in our group had never done any kind of multisport event before. I experienced none of the fear or nerves of my first time, but the newbies reminded me how I'd felt just two years before. My goal this time: have fun. The result: I had a fabulous time and I achieved a personal record for the event.

How different would our FB50 Challenge be if, instead, it had been "Fittest by 30"? As I approached 30, I undertook physical activity with one primary purpose in mind: to lose weight (or maintain it if I'd hit my "goal" in recent days or weeks). I had a tough resistance training routine at the gym. Sometimes, to get my cardio in, I spent hours with a good novel on the stationary bike. I walked hard and far every day. My approach has evolved 180 degrees from that time.

The FB50 Challenge put me in touch with my fun side—no more punishing routines whose only goal is fitness. In those last months of the challenge, I learned to push myself with different motives in mind, mostly out of curiosity about what my body could do. I'd never been a runner, let alone a runner with goals. But I threw myself into that last summer of training leading up to my 50th aiming for a sub-65-minute 10K running time, plus the ambitious dream of completing those Olympic distance triathlons in less than 3 hours and 30 minutes. I came close to the sub-65 10K. I had my best finish, 3:44, at Lakeside. I missed my sub-3:30, but hey, two weeks before that I had zipped around the Nevada desert on a gearless bicycle with back-pedal brakes, off the grid at Burning Man.

We all know that platitude about aging as a state of mind. Despite the prominent and public goal of achieving my fittest by 50, that looming birthday didn't dominate my thoughts at all that summer. The triathlons and the training required for them nudged aside all thoughts of aging.

Past the midpoint of my life, who could deny the astonishing awesomeness of the last year of the FB50 Challenge? That voice in my head could try: *You're past the prime of youth. Maybe you're in good condition now, but you've peaked. It has to be downhill from here, right? How much better can you expect to get if you're already 50?*

When we started, I didn't want to run, never mind run faster. Now? Half marathon, anyone? When we started, triathlon was not even in the picture! At the outset of our challenge, I thought the bod pod would be a good way to measure my progress. Now, screw the bod pod. And when we started, I didn't think of myself as an athlete at all. Now, I feel comfortable with the idea that I'm an athlete. Elite athletes aren't the only athletes, and not all athletes have to be champions.

I see an older, wiser me. At this time of life, I aim for strength in my weight training, not a particular aesthetic. I'm also okay with doing less when I feel like it. Truth be told, I am stronger, faster, fitter, more energetic, and most importantly, *happier* than I used to be.

I'm excited about mid-life. As Sam says, "40 is the old age of youth and 50 is the youth of old age." Here's to our newfound youth!

Sam Pedals Right Past 50

There are no truly convenient deaths. I had thought after the deaths of my father- and mother-in-law during the challenge that I was done with death for a while. That was my plan but death reminds us how fruitless plans are, really. Everything changes, and nothing stays the same. While Tracy and I were writing this book, my own father's health was failing as he faced a diagnosis of esophageal cancer, and he died the year after our challenge ended.

With my 50th birthday behind me, I just kept on moving. And with the growing blog community and my fitness friends, I never felt that I was in it alone. There was no temptation, even during the worst of things, to throw in the towel. Since the challenge ended, I've been working with a cycling coach, and the winter after I turned 50 I went to my first-ever winter training camp in the hills of South Carolina. Pre-season training camp is where you go to get a jump on the outdoor cycling season and travel south not for the beaches or the scenery, but to train with other cyclists who want to be fast when the outdoor season begins at home. There was no bus riding along behind us to pick us up when we'd had enough, like on the cycling holidays I'd done. There was no tour guide with snacks. Unlike those holidays, I did not get to take very many photos. Instead, we rode fast all morning and got back in to camp just after lunch. There was napping, more eating, and then early to bed. We repeated that each day and I got faster on the hills as the week progressed. It was a brand-new experience for me that challenged me physically. I'm riding with the fast group now with my cycling coach, and while I get dropped (that means "left behind") when we do intervals, I'm a lot faster than I was last year when I stuck with his intermediate riders.

But the year after the challenge wasn't all about speed. It seems that having ridden my bike from Toronto to Montreal once, I needed to do it again. My second bike rally ride was with one of the blog's regular guests, Susan Tarshis. Together we rode our bikes from Toronto to Montreal, with the Friends for Life Bike Rally, to raise funds for people living with HIV/AIDS in Toronto. I've done quite a few organized century rides and Gran Fondos too (Wikipedia describes a Gran Fondo as "a type of long-distance road bicycle ride originating in Italy in 1970," and adds that it "roughly translates into English as 'Big Ride' "). The year after the challenge I branched out and bought a snazzy new road bike and a matching snazzy new cyclocross bike. It's fun to fly on the grass and the gravel. I haven't mastered the art of bunny hopping (that's when you jump with the bike) yet, but that skill is on my list of things to try. I've also tried fat biking—those are bikes with the really wide tires you ride through the snow. Fifty isn't slowing me down at all. The summer I approached 51 even saw me stepping back into the pool. I'm getting help with my swimming from the community of feminist fitness friends that's gathered around our blog, and I'm thinking I might try triathlon again next summer. I also bought my own lightweight canoe for camping and canoeing holidays, adding to my repertoire of active vacations. A new puppy brought a new purpose to running, as well. I taught our little lab-husky, Cheddar, to run along at my side. Amid all of life's ups and downs, my fitness activities were a source of stress relief, the place I found friends and community, and they added lots of joy to my life.

Happy birthday to us: fit, feminist, over 50, and fine with that!

NOTES

CHAPTER 2 *Older and Wiser*

1. Krista Scott Dixon, "In Praise of Older Women," Stumptuous, February 2012, www.stumptuous.com/rant-63-february-2012-in-praise-of-older-women.

2. "Older Athletes' Age in Fitness Terms 'Astounding,' Doctor Says," *CBC News*, July 2, 2015, www.cbc.ca/news/health/older-athletes-age-in-fitness-terms-astounding-doctor-says-1.3136319.

3. Ian Sample, "Old Before Your Time? People Age at Wildly Different Rates, Study Confirms," *The Guardian,* July 6, 2015, www.theguardian.com/science/2015/jul/06/old-before-your-time-people-age-at-wildly-different-rates-study-confirms.

4. Nelson Rice, "Exercise Makes You Smarter as You Age," *Runner's World,* June 29, 2015, www.runnersworld.com/health/exercise-makes-you-smarter-as-you-age.

5. Gretchen Reynolds, *The First 20 Minutes: Surprising Science Reveals How We Can Exercise Better, Train Smarter, Live Longer* (New York: Penguin, 2012).

6. Amy Noser and Virgil Zeigler-Hill, "Investing in the Ideal: Does Objectified Body Consciousness Mediate the Association between Appearance Contingent Self-Worth and Appearance Self-Esteem in Women?" *Body Image* 11, no. 2 (2014): 119–25, doi:10.1016/j.bodyim.2013.11.006.

7. Selene Yeager, "Be Proud of Your Body," *Bicycling,* July 22, 2015, www.bicycling.com/training/motivation/be-proud-your-body.

8. Check out your fitness age at the World Fitness Level website: www.worldfitnesslevel.org.

9. Cristin D. Runfola, Ann Von Holle, Christine M. Peat, Danielle A. Gagne, Kimberly A. Brownley, Sara M. Hofmeier, and Cynthia M. Bulik, "Characteristics of Women with Body Size Satisfaction at Midlife: Results of the Gender and Body Image (GABI) Study," *Journal of Women & Aging* 25, no. 4 (2013): 287–304, doi:10.1080/08952841.2013.816215.

CHAPTER 3 *Feminist Fitness Is for Everyone*

1. Katty Kay and Claire Shipman, "The Confidence Gap," *The Atlantic,* May 2014, www.theatlantic.com/magazine/archive/2014/05/the-confidence-gap/359815/.

2. Gretchen Reynolds, "The Benefits of Exercising Outdoors," *New York Times,* February 21, 2013, well.blogs.nytimes.com/2013/02/21/the-benefits-of-exercising-outdoors/.

3. "Benefits of Outdoor Exercise Confirmed," *Science Daily,* February 5, 2011, www.sciencedaily.com/releases/2011/02/110204130607.htm. The study referenced there is J. Thompson Coon, K. Boddy, K. Stein, R. Whear, J. Barton, and M.H. Depledge, "Does Participating in Physical Activity in Outdoor Natural Environments Have a Greater Effect on Physical and Mental Wellbeing Than Physical Activity Indoors? A Systematic Review," *Environmental Science & Technology* 45, no. 5 (2011): 1761–72, doi: 10.1021/es102947t.

4. Michelle Segar, Jennifer M. Taber, Heather Patrick, Chan L. Thai, and April Oh, "Rethinking Physical Activity Communication: Using Focus Groups to Understand Women's Goals, Values, and Beliefs to Improve Public Health," *BMC Public Health* 17 (2017), doi:10.1186/s12889-017-4361-1.

5. Jan Eickmeier, "Few Middle-Aged Women Are Happy with Their Body Size: The Ones Most Likely to Be Are Highly Active," *Runner's World,* October 18, 2013, www.runnersworld.com/newswire/few-middle-aged-women-are-happy-with-their-body-size.

6. Selene Yeager, "Be Proud of Your Body," *Bicycling,* July 22, 2015, www.bicycling.com/training/motivation/be-proud-your-body.

7. Ann J. Cahill, "What (Feminist) Self-Defense Courses Can Do," Fit Is a Feminist Issue, June 25, 2015, fitisafeministissue.com/2015/06/25/what-feminist-self-defense-courses-can-do-guest-post/.

8. Jean Fain, "Eve Ensler on Cancer, Her Body, and the 'Body of the World,' " *Huffington Post,* April 26, 2013, www.huffingtonpost.com/jean-fain-licsw-msw/eve-ensler-cancer_b_3163527.html.

CHAPTER 5 *Sure, Let's Get Fit, but Fit for What?*

1. Miriam E. Nelson, Maria A. Fiatarone, Christina M. Morganti, Isaiah Trice, Robert A. Greenberg, and William J. Evans, "Effects of High-Intensity Strength Training on Multiple Risk Factors for Osteoporotic Fractures: A Randomized Controlled Trial," *JAMA* 272, no. 24 (1994): 1909–14, doi:10.1001/jama.1994.03520240037038.

2. See Sophia Breene, "13 Mental Health Benefits of Exercise," *Huffington Post,* March 27, 2013, www.huffingtonpost.com/2013/03/27/mental-health-benefits-exercise_n_2956099.html.

CHAPTER 6 *Love Your Body Now*

1. "This Girl Can: New Campaign Urges More Women to Get Active," BBC *Sport,* January 12, 2015, www.bbc.com/sport/get-inspired/30743750.

2. Simon MacMichael, "Nine in Ten Women over 30 Scared to Take Part in Outdoor Exercise, Says Mental Health Charity Mind," *Road,* April 24, 2012, road.cc/content/news/57107-nine-ten-women-over-30-scared-take-part-outdoor-exercise-says-mental-health.

3. Natasha Hinde, "Women Are Running on Treadmills in Sheds Because They 'Fear Being Judged', Government Report Reveals," *Huffington Post,* March 25, 2015, www.huffingtonpost.co.uk/2015/03/25/women-not-working-out-fear-of-being-judged_n_6938448.html.

4. Michael R. Lowe, Tanja V. E. Kral, and Karen Miller-Kovach, "Weight-Loss Maintenance 1, 2 and 5 Years after Successful Completion of a Weight-Loss Programme," *British Journal of Nutrition* 99, no. 4 (2008): 925–30, doi:10.1017/s0007114507862416.

5. Erin Fothergill, Juen Guo, Lilian Howard, Jennifer C. Kerns, Nicolas D. Knuth, Robert Brychta, et al., "Persistent Metabolic Adaptation 6 Years after 'The Biggest Loser' Competition," *Obesity* 24, no. 8 (2016): 1612–19, doi:10.1002/oby.21538.

6. "10 Principles of Intuitive Eating," Intuitive Eating, www.intuitiveeating.org/10-principles-of-intuitive-eating.

7. Ann Cahill, "Getting to My Fighting Weight," *Hypatia* 25, no. 2 (Spring 2010): 491.

CHAPTER 8 *The FB50 Challenge: Six Months to One Year*

1. Rod Cedaro, "Learn to Master the Bike-Run Transition," Active.com, n.d., www.active.com/duathlon/articles/learn-to-master-the-bike-to-run-transition.

2. Thomas Hurka, "Hypocrisy: Not All It's Cracked Down to Be," reprinted in *Principles: Short Essays on Ethics* (Toronto: Harcourt Brace Canada, 1993), 264.

3. John Seabrook, "Feel No Pain: Rowing's Unlikely Hero Has Dedicated His Life to the Most Gruelling Sport," *The New Yorker,* July 22, 1996, www.johnseabrook.com/feel-no-pain/.

4. Charlotte Hilton Andersen, "25 Most Deceiving Exercises (They Tone More than You Think!)" *Shape,* n.d., www.shape.com/fitness/workouts/25-most-deceiving-exercises-they-tone-more-you-think.

CHAPTER 9 *Hey, Girl! The Feminization of Fitness*

1. Erin Ellis, "Women-Only Section of Vancouver Gym to Be Phased Out," *Vancouver Sun,* September 9, 2014, www.vancouversun.com/health/Steve+Nash+Downtown+Vancouver+eliminates+women+only+section/9365453/story.html.

2. "Why Is Race for Life a Women-Only Event?" Cancer Research UK Race for Life Facebook page, January 7, 2013, www.facebook.com/notes/cancer-research-uk-race-for-life/why-is-race-for-life-a-women-only-event/10151166317152003/.

CHAPTER 10 *Exercise in Everyday Life*

1. Wyatt Myers, "NEAT Exercises for Couch Potatoes," Everyday Health, July 11, 2012, www.everydayhealth.com/fitness/neat-exercises-for-couch-potatoes.aspx.

2. "London Transport Workers Study," Heart Attack Prevention: A History of Cardiovascular Disease Epidemiology, University of Minnesota, n.d., www.epi.umn.edu/cvdepi/study-synopsis/london-transport-workers-study/.

3. D. D. Dunlop, J. Song, E. K. Arnston, P. A. Semanik, J. Lee, R. W. Chang, J. M. Hootman, "Sedentary Time in US Older Adults Associated with Disability in Activities of Daily Living Independent of Physical Activity," *Journal of Physical Activity & Health* 12, no. 1 (2015): 93–101.

4. Kathryn Hayes, "Teen Girls 'Risk Hearts Sitting for 20 Hours a Day'," *Irish Independent,* May 15, 2014, www.independent.ie/lifestyle/health/teen-girls-risk-hearts-sitting-for-20-hours-a-day-30276102.html.

5. Nancy Clark, "Sedentary Athletes: Sitting and Weighting," My Net Diary, March 1, 2011, www.mynetdiary.com/sedentary-athletes-sitting-weighting.html.

6. Gretchen Reynolds, "For Weight Loss, Less Exercise May Be More," *New York Times,* September 19, 2012, well.blogs.nytimes.com/2012/09/19/is-30-minutes-of-daily-exercise-a-sweet-spot-for-weight-loss/.

7. Colin McSwiggen, "Against Chairs," *Jacobin,* no. 6, April 22, 2012, www.jacobinmag.com/2012/04/against-chairs/.

8. Kathleen Hale, "Why Sitting Is Bad for You and How to Avoid It," March 23, 2016, Livestrong, www.livestrong.com/article/1011295-sitting-bad-avoid/.

9. See American Heart Association, "Taking public transportation instead of driving linked with better health," *ScienceDaily*, November 8, 2015, www.sciencedaily.com/releases/2015/11/151108124754.htm.

10. Michael Grothaus, "Here's What the iPhone Reveals about Suburbanites vs. City Dwellers," *Engadget*, January 9, 2014, www.engadget.com/2014/01/09/heres-what-the-iphone-reveals-about-suburbanites-vs-city-dwelle/.

11. Tara Parker-Pope, "The Pedometer Test: Americans Take Fewer Steps," *New York Times,* October 19, 2010, well.blogs.nytimes.com/2010/10/19/the-pedometer-test-americans-take-fewer-steps/.

CHAPTER 11 *Let's Move! Taking Care of Our Cardio Health*

1. Linda Baker, "How to Get More Bicyclists on the Road," *Scientific American,* October 1, 2009, www.scientificamerican.com/article/getting-more-bicyclists-on-the-road/.

2. Jan Garrard, Susan Handy, and Jennifer Dill, "Women and Cycling," in John Pucher and Ralph Buehler, eds., *City Cycling* (Cambridge, Mass.: MIT Press, 2012).

3. "The Top 5 Benefits of Cycling," *Harvard Health Letter,* August 2016, www.health.harvard.edu/staying-healthy/the-top-5-benefits-of-cycling.

4. For a list of the mental health benefits of cycling, see Hilary Angus, "Pedaling towards Happiness: 7 Mental Health Benefits of Riding Bikes," *Momentum,* March 29, 2016, momentummag.com/mental-health-benefits-of-cycling/.

CHAPTER 13 *Muscles, Strength, and Mobility*

1. "How to Do a Deadlift," *WikiHow*, accessed July 5, 2017, www.wikihow.com/Do-a-Deadlift.

2. "Falling in Aikido," Aikido Centers, accessed July 5, 2017, www.aikidocenters.com/Falling-in-Aikido.shtml.

CHAPTER 14 *Families and Fitness*

1. Associated Press, "Kids Less Fit than Parents Worldwide," *CBC News*, November 19, 2013, www.cbc.ca/m/touch/health/story/1.2432307.

2. K.J. Dell'Antonia, "Dance Class: An 'Activity' That Isn't Very Active," *New York Times,* May 22, 2015, mobile.nytimes.com/blogs/parenting/2015/05/22/dance-class-an-activity-that-isnt-very-active/.

3. Bridget Yard, "Effects of Poor Physical Literacy in Children Carry into Adulthood," *CBC News*, January 28, 2015, www.cbc.ca/news/canada/new-brunswick/effects-of-poor-physical-literacy-in-children-carry-into-adulthood-1.2933485.

4. Sue Y.S. Kimm, Nancy W. Glynn, Andrea M. Kriska, Bruce A. Barton, Shari S. Kronsberg, Stephen R. Daniels, et al., "Decline in Physical Activity in Black Girls and White Girls during Adolescence," *New England Journal of Medicine* 347, no. 10 (2002): 709–15, doi: 10.1056/NEJMoa003277; "Teenage Girls Sit or Lie Down for 19 Hours a Day—but What Effect Is It Having on Their Heart?" *The Journal* (Ireland), May 15, 2014, www.thejournal.ie/university-of-limerick-sitting-down-heart-1465802-May2014/.

5. Statistics Canada, *Sport Participation in Canada, 2005* (Ottawa: Statistics Canada, Culture, Tourism and the Centre for Educational Statistics Division, 2008).

CHAPTER 15 *Keeping It Realistic: Achieving a Sustainable Routine*

1. Dick Talens, "The Myth of Willpower and 'Eat Less, Move More,' " Musings of a Dick, March 21, 2013, sett.com/dicktalens/the-myth-of-willpower-and-eat-less-move-more.

2. Juliette Kellow, "Turn Housework into a Workout," www.weightlossresources. co.uk/exercise/tips/housework_workouts.htm.

3. See Duncan Haughey, "SMART goals," Project SMART, accessed July 5, 2017, www.projectsmart.co.uk/smart-goals.php.

4. Sam Brennan, "My Whole Life Is Workout Time," Fit Is a Feminist Issue, January 16, 2013, fitisafeministissue.com/2013/01/16/ my-whole-life-is-workout-time/.

5. Amby Burfoot, "New Research: Big Benefits from Running 5 Miles a Week," *Runners' World,* July 29, 2014, www.runnersworld.com/newswire/ new-research-big-benefits-from-running-5-miles-a-week.

CHAPTER 16 *The FB50 Challenge: The Last Six Months*

1. Stephanie Pearl-McPhee, "These Words Are Like Birds," August 5, 2014, www.yarnharlot.ca/2014/08/these-words-are-like-birds/.

2. Stephanie Pearl-McPhee, "Thank You," July 26, 2014, www.yarnharlot. ca/2014/07/.

About the Authors

SAMANTHA BRENNAN, PhD, is Dean of the College of Arts at the University of Guelph, President of the Canadian Philosophical Association, and a co-founder and co-editor of *Feminist Philosophy Quarterly*.

TRACY ISAACS, PhD, is Associate Dean (Academic) in the Faculty of Arts and Humanities and a professor in the Departments of Philosophy and of Women's Studies and Feminist Research at Western University. *Fit at Mid-Life* is her second non-fiction book.